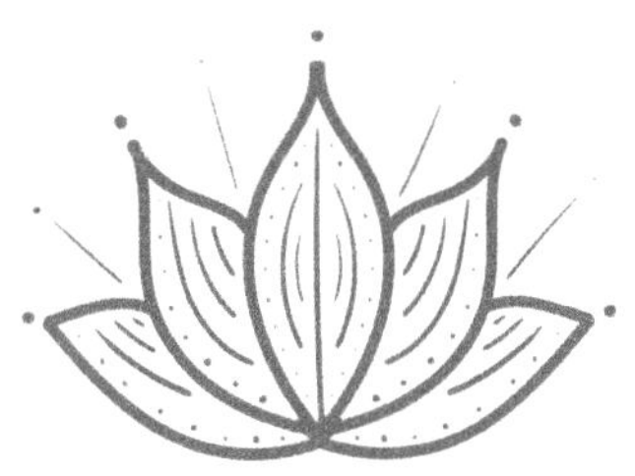

CHAIR YOGA FOR SENIORS OVER 60

Lose Weight while Gaining Mobility, Strength & Balance in Just Minutes a Day with Gentle Exercises.

Simon Joy

As part of your commitment to improving mobility, strength, balance, and embarking on a weight loss journey, we're excited to present you with some exclusive bonus content.

Let me ask you a few questions.

- Wouldn't it be amazing to feel the rejuvenating effects of clean eating coupled with your yoga routine?
- Are you ready to challenge yourself and witness a remarkable transformation in your strength and mobility?
- How about enhancing your yoga practice with guided audio routines, making it easier and more enjoyable to stay on track?

If you answered **YES** at least of one of these questions, then you don't want to miss this special occasion.

Scanning the QR Code below you will have instant access to 3 different Bonuses

1. 28-Day Chair Yoga Fitness Challenge
2. 15-Day Clean Eating Challenge
3. 3Audio Routines

TABLE OF CONTENTS

It's no secret that regular physical activity is key to maintaining and improving health, especially as we age. However, the Centers for Disease Control and Prevention (CDC) reports that less than 30% of adults aged 65 and older are meeting the recommended guidelines for physical activity. This lack of exercise can lead to increased risks of falls, cognitive decline, and chronic diseases such as heart disease and diabetes.

If you're eager to join that health-conscious 30% and enhance not only your physical but also your mental health, "Chair Yoga for Seniors" is the perfect guide for you. This book is specifically designed to help you lose weight, gain mobility, strength, and balance through gentle, effective exercises that can be done in just minutes a day.

Yoga is renowned for its wide range of benefits for seniors, including increased flexibility, stronger bones, and reduced stress. However, traditional yoga can be daunting for those with mobility issues or chronic pain. Chair yoga offers a wonderful solution. By using a chair for support, either sitting or standing, chair yoga adapts traditional yoga into a gentle form that is accessible to almost anyone, regardless of age, ability, or fitness level.

Here's why chair yoga is an excellent exercise choice:

- **Suitable for Almost Anyone:** Chair yoga is ideal for those who have difficulty with traditional exercises, providing an accessible way to maintain fitness and mobility.

- **Gentle and Low-Impact:** This low-impact workout is kind to the joints, perfect for those dealing with arthritis, mobility concerns, or other medical conditions. It gently improves flexibility and balance without straining the body.

- **Weight Loss and Improved Circulation:** Along with aiding weight loss, the movements in chair yoga enhance circulation, reducing muscle stiffness and the likelihood of falls, thereby boosting overall mobility.

- **Stress Reduction**: Incorporating breathing and meditation, chair yoga is effective in lowering stress and anxiety, contributing to better mental health.

- **Convenience:** Easily practiced at home or in a group, chair yoga is a convenient option for seniors with limited mobility or transportation.

Our book, "Chair Yoga for Seniors," offers a safe and accessible approach to traditional yoga. It is designed to fit into your daily routine effortlessly, leading to improved health and well-being. We provide all the necessary tools, techniques, and routines to improve balance and mobility, helping you reap the benefits of this ancient practice in a modern, senior-friendly format. So, let's embark on this journey together and explore the transformative power of chair yoga for seniors.

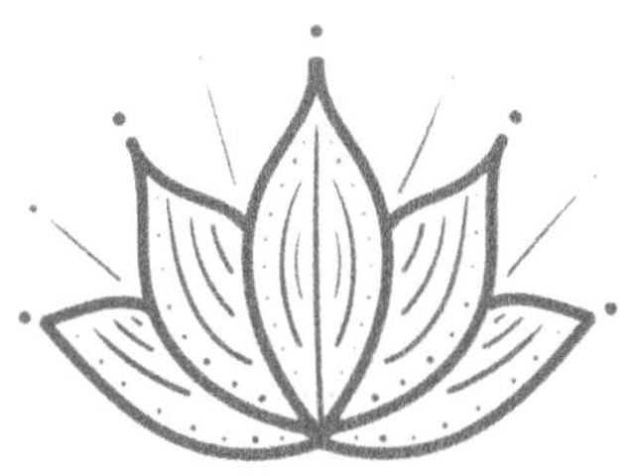

Integrating yoga practice into your daily lifestyle can potentially enhance your overall well-being as it can positively impact your physical and cognitive health, foster a sense of calmness, and diminish stress levels. Consider the following strategies to incorporate yoga practice into your routine effectively.

- Start small: One approach to easing into yoga for beginners is by commencing with brief, uncomplicated routines that can be seamlessly incorporated into your everyday schedule.

- Even just a few minutes of yoga in the morning or before bed can be beneficial. Remember to listen to your body and begin slowly, increasing the length and intensity of your practice as you become more comfortable.

- Establish a dedicated area for practicing at home: A suitable area for practicing yoga could consist of a separate and allotted room in your residence or a designated corner within an existing room. Establishing a designated area for yoga within one's living space can enhance the consistency of practice and foster a sense of calm and serenity within the home environment.

- Establish a consistent practice schedule: Endeavor to designate a particular time daily to engage in your yoga routine. Incorporating this into your daily regimen can promote consistency.

- Incorporate the core tenets of yoga into your everyday behaviors and thinking patterns. This encompasses upholding ethical principles, being conscious of your thoughts and behaviors, and harmonizing your lifestyle with your values and those around you. In addition, incorporating a nutritious and well-rounded diet, engaging in mindfulness techniques, and prioritizing self-care and relaxation can also be beneficial.

SCIENTIFICALLY PROVEN BENEFITS

A growing body of scientific research suggests chair yoga can offer a range of physical and mental health benefits. Here are some of the key findings:

- A 2011 study [1] in the Evidence-based Complementary and Alternative Medicine Journal showed that an 8-week yoga program effectively reduced blood pressure, stress, anxiety, and sleep disturbances in senior women, offering a safe intervention for overall wellness.

- Research in the International Journal of Environmental Research and Public Health (2021) advocates promoting chair-based exercises to improve strength and balance, countering the effects of physical inactivity in older adults. This study [2] noted significant improvements in balance, gait speed, and grip strength among participants.

- An older adult yoga program, as reported in a 2009 article in the same journal, proved both achievable and beneficial. Over three months, participants improved in exercise self-efficacy and cardiometabolic risk factors, demonstrating the program's holistic health benefits.

- A 2016 study [4] published in the National Library of Medicine found that seniors with lower extremity osteoarthritis experienced reduced pain and fatigue following an 8-week chair yoga program, also noting improved mobility.

- A 2013 study [5] concluded that yoga contributed to a significant reduction in blood pressure in individuals with prehypertension or hypertension, particularly when combining postures, meditation, and breathing techniques.

Kim E. Innes, and Terry Kit Selfe. "The Effects of a Gentle Yoga Program on Sleep, Mood, and Blood Pressure in Older Women with Restless Legs Syndrome (RLS): A Preliminary Randomized Controlled Trial" Evidence-Based Complementary and Alternative Medicine, vol. 2012, 2012. doi:10.1155/2012/294058

Klempel N, Blackburn NE, McMullan IL, Wilson JJ, Smith L, Cunningham C, O'Sullivan R, Caserotti P, Tully MA. The Effect of Chair-Based Exercise on Physical Function in Older Adults: A Systematic Review and Meta-Analysis. Int J Environ Res Public Health. 2021 Feb 16;18(4):1902. doi: 10.3390/ijerph18041902. PMID: 33669357; PMCID: PMC7920319.

Kyeongra Yang, Lisa M. Bernardo, Susan M. Sereika, Molly B. Conroy, Judy Balk, and Lora E. Burke. "Utilization of 3-Month Yoga Program for Adults at High Risk for Type 2 Diabetes: A Pilot Study" Evidence-Based Complementary and Alternative Medicine, vol. 2011, 2009. doi:10.1093/ecam/nep117

Park J, McCaffrey R, Newman D, Liehr P, Ouslander JG. A Pilot Randomized Controlled Trial of the Effects of Chair Yoga on Pain and Physical Function Among Community-Dwelling Older Adults with Lower Extremity Osteoarthritis. J Am Geriatr Soc. 2017 Mar;65(3):592-597. doi: 10.1111/jgs.14717. Epub 2016 Dec 23. PMID: 28008603; PMCID: PMC5357158.

Marshall Hagins, Rebecca States, Terry Selfe, and Kim Innes. "Effectiveness of Yoga for Hypertension: Systematic Review and Meta-Analysis" Evidence-Based Complementary and Alternative Medicine, vol. 2013, 2013. doi:10.1155/2013/64983

ARE THERE ANY CONTRAINDICATIONS?

While chair yoga is suitable for most seniors as it is a low-impact form of exercise, there may be some contraindications to practicing, depending on an individual's health and medical conditions. Here are some potential contraindications to keep in mind:

- Recent surgeries: If you've recently had surgery or are recovering from an injury, it's crucial to get approval from your healthcare provider before starting or resuming any exercise program.

- Severe joint pain: Those experiencing significant joint pain should consider modifying poses or avoiding certain movements altogether. Pay close attention to your body's signals to understand your limits.

- Balance issues: For individuals with severe balance issues or dizziness, some standing poses may pose a risk. In such cases, focus primarily on seated poses to ensure safety.

- Cardiovascular issues: If you have a history of heart disease or high blood pressure, consult your doctor before beginning chair yoga or any new exercise routine. Tailoring your practice to accommodate your cardiovascular health is important.

- Respiratory issues: People with respiratory conditions, like COPD, should adjust their practice accordingly, especially when it comes to breathing exercises. It might be necessary to avoid certain practices or modify them under the guidance of a healthcare professional.

Later in this book, detailed contraindications for each pose, along with possible variations, will be provided. However, consulting with a medical professional is paramount before starting any new exercise regimen, including chair yoga, especially if you have pre-existing health conditions or concerns.

WHAT DO YOU NEED TO START?

One of the great things about chair yoga is that it requires minimal equipment or special tools, making it an accessible form of exercise for many people. Here are some of the tools you might need or want to have on hand to practice chair yoga:

- A chair: The most important tool for chair yoga is a sturdy, stable chair without wheels. Ideally, it should be a chair with a straight back and no armrests, but armrests can be used for some poses.

- Comfortable clothing: Wearing comfortable, non-restrictive clothes that allow for a broad motion range is essential. Ideal clothing is loose-fitting, permeable clothing.

- Yoga mat or non-slip surface: While not strictly necessary, a yoga mat or non-slip surface can be helpful to provide extra grip and stability during standing poses.

- Blocks, straps, or blankets: These accessories can be used to change or simplify poses. For example, a blanket can be folded to provide extra support under the hips, while a block can be used to bring the ground closer in seated poses.

- Timer: Sometimes, it is useful to have a timer or a clock to time your exercises.

- Water bottle: Each kind of activity requires you to stay hydrated, so it stands to reason to have a water bottle with you.

To summarize, chair yoga is a low-maintenance exercise that can be done practically anywhere. You can begin a gentle, effective yoga practice that can help improve your physical and mental health with nothing more than a chair and comfortable clothing.

THINGS TO KEEP IN MIND

As with any physical activity, listening to your body and respecting your limits is crucial in chair yoga. Always modify or ease up on a pose if it causes discomfort or pain. Here are key practices to ensure a beneficial yoga experience:

- Deep Breathing: Maintain deep, consistent breathing to stay composed and focused. As your breathing skills improve, you'll find you can deepen your poses and enhance your practice.

- Diverse Poses: Experiment with various poses to engage different muscle groups and achieve a comprehensive workout.

- Injury Prevention Tips:

    - Warm-Up and Cool-Down: Incorporate warm-up and cool-down exercises along with traditional asanas to prepare and restore your body.

    - Posture Awareness: Pay attention to your posture for better alignment. Sit up straight and engage your core muscles to stabilize your spine.

- Nutrition's Role: Don't underestimate the importance of a healthy diet, which is an integral part of chair yoga. Proper nutrition provides the energy and nutrients necessary for physical activity and overall health. It can also improve mood, reduce stress, and assist in maintaining a healthy weight, especially if you focus on a balanced diet low in processed foods.

- Using Props: Utilize props like blocks, straps, or blankets to modify poses and enhance accessibility. Props can provide support and help you ease into poses more comfortably.

- Take Breaks: If you feel tired, don't hesitate to modify your pose, or take a break. Paying attention to your body's signals and avoiding overexertion is essential.

Remember, the goal of chair yoga is not only physical improvement but also mental and emotional well-being. Gradually build up your practice and allow your body to adapt at its own pace.

CHAPTER 2: HOW TO STRUCTURE YOUR CHAIR YOGA ROUTINE

One key factor that makes a chair yoga session successful is structuring the practice in a way tailored to the individual's needs and abilities. In this chapter, we will discuss how to use this book to structure a yoga session and how to effectively structure a chair yoga session using our 5-step routine.

Step 1. Breathing

Start with a brief period of breath-centered mindfulness. This helps in easing your mental state and preparing your body for the exercises to come.

Step 2. Set Your Intention

After about a minute of deep breathing, pause to set a clear intention for your session. Whether it's enhancing balance, increasing flexibility, or alleviating stress, having a specific goal can help focus your practice and boost motivation. During your practice, keep this intention in mind to maintain focus.

While formulating your intention for the practice, you must contemplate the desired outcomes you wish to accomplish. Would you like to enhance your balance, boost your flexibility, or alleviate stress? One can effectively curate suitable poses and sequences for their regimen by keeping their objectives in mind.

Concentrating the mind, establishing a precise objective for the routine, and outlining a goal-oriented path for the activity can aid in the process. Having a well-defined objective can foster high levels of motivation and engagement throughout the session. Moreover, articulating your purpose can facilitate the establishment of a clear trajectory for the session, streamlining the progression of the various poses and routines more systematically and purposefully.

The goals of a chair yoga session may consist of:

- "My objective is to enhance my equilibrium and steadiness."
- "My objective is to promote an atmosphere of serenity and peacefulness."
- "I possess a high level of physical strength and flexibility."

Finally, we come to the "Asanas", as we call physical posture or pose in the practice of yoga. Each asana is designed to target specific areas of the body, promote flexibility and strength, and support overall health and well-being.

"Asana" is also sometimes used more broadly to refer to the overall practice of yoga, which includes not only physical postures but also meditation, breathing techniques, ethical guidelines, and other elements of the practice. In this book, when we refer to "Asana" we are talking about any physical posture inside this Yoga Guide.

Tailor-made routines in the following chapters provide step-by-step instructions. Remember to listen to your body and move fluidly from one pose to the next.

Step 4. Pranayama

It is important to include Pranayama, or yogic breathing techniques at the end of a yoga practice because it can help to promote a sense of balance and calm. In **Chapter 3**, we will explain some useful Pranayama techniques for integrating the benefits of your yoga practice into your daily life.

Step 5. Relaxation (Savasana), Gratitude & Meditation

To finish chair yoga practice, it's important to take a few minutes to allow your body and mind to fully absorb the benefits of the practice, and to bring your breathing and heart rate back to a resting state. Here are a few steps you can follow to end your chair yoga practice:

Seated Relaxation or Savasana.

Chair Savasana is a relaxation technique that is often used to end a yoga session and is generally performed while lying on your back. However, in chair yoga, you can modify the pose to be done in a seated position.

You can experience several advantages from practicing Chair Savasana, including better sleep, a reduction in tension and anxiety, and an overall boost in emotions of well-being. Moreover, it can enhance circulation, relieve soreness, and generally improve mobility and flexibility. Additionally, Chair Savasana can help to improve focus and concentration, making it a great way to end a yoga session.

Gratitude

Once you finish "Chair Savasana," express gratitude for your body, practice, and anything else that comes to mind. This approach can significantly shift one's perspective and promote positive attitudes.

Some examples:

- I am grateful for the physiological capabilities of my body, encompassing its aptitude for physical activity and breathing patterns.
- I am grateful for the level of commitment I have shown in completing the task.
- I am grateful for my dedication to completing my daily practice.

MEDITATION

You may find engaging in a brief seated meditation beneficial, directing your focus towards your breath or a specific intention.

It is imperative to acknowledge that meditation is a personal endeavor and there is no right or wrong way to do it. The secret is to determine a viable strategy that aligns with your requirements and consistently upholds adherence. Integrating a regular meditation practice into one's daily routine, even if done for short durations, can improve one's holistic well-being.

Here are a few fundamental measures to commence:

1. Find a quiet, comfortable place.
2. Set a timer for a few minutes, gradually increasing the duration.
3. Start with deep breaths to relax.
4. Choose a focus point for your meditation.
5. Gently bring your mind back whenever it wanders.
6. After meditating, take a moment to notice any changes in your well-being.

Keep in mind that developing your meditation skills takes effort and patience. Try to meditate at the same time every day and incorporate it into your routine on a regular basis. With frequent practice, you could start to feel better physically and emotionally.

By following these steps, you can bring your chair yoga practice to a peaceful and mindful close, helping to promote a sense of relaxation and well-being that can last throughout your day.

TIPS TO A BETTER PRACTICE:

- Make sure that your chair is comfortable and supportive.
- Try counting your breaths or repeating a word or sound (called typically mantra) to help you focus if you have difficulties focusing or keeping your mind from wandering.
- It is important to practice Chair Savasana in a quiet, distraction free environment.
- Express gratitude in advance for all the benefits that you will get from your daily practice.
- Express gratitude to yourself always.
- If you have balance issues when performing a pose, look at a fixed point, breathe deep and start again.

In summary, structuring a chair yoga session involves assessing your physical abilities and limitations, identifying your goals, choosing appropriate poses and sequences, considering timing and environment, and approaching the practice with a positive attitude. By following the guidelines in this book and creating a personalized routine, you will be well on your way to a successful chair yoga practice.

CHAPTER 3: CHAIR YOGA STEP BY STEP INSTRUCTIONS

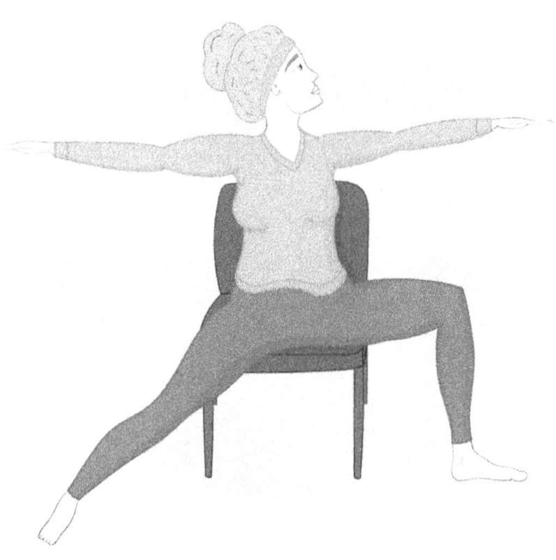

In this chapter, we delve into a variety of chair yoga poses aimed at improving strength, flexibility, balance, and relaxation. These poses are tailored to be accessible to practitioners of all abilities and can be easily modified to accommodate individual needs and limitations..

Asanas For All

Whether you're new to yoga or an experienced practitioner, these chair yoga poses offer a safe and effective way to incorporate yoga into your daily life. They are suitable for people of all ages and fitness levels.

This foundational pose is the starting point for most chair yoga routines, promoting good posture, spine alignment, and a calm, focused mind. It is particularly accessible for seniors and individuals with mobility challenges.

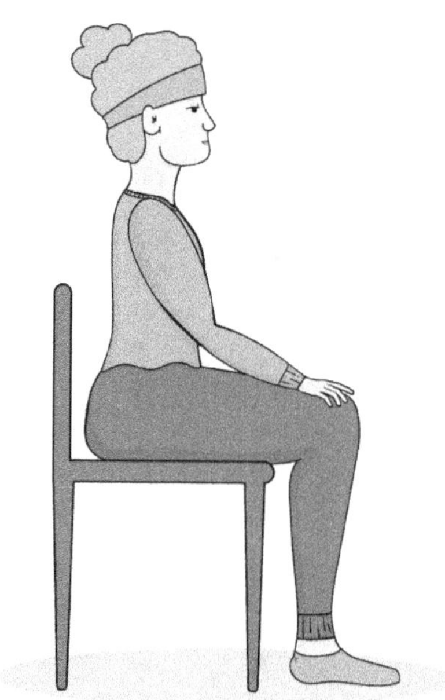

Limitations:

Ideal for those who find it difficult to get down to or up from the floor.

Benefits:

- Encourages good posture and spine alignment.
- Fosters a calm and focused mind.

1. Sit on your chair, straighten your spine, and place your feet firmly on the ground.

2. Place your hand on your thighs, palm facing up or down, whatever makes you most comfortable.

3. Inhale deeply using your nose while closing your eyes: As you inhale, fill your lungs with air and expand your belly. Count to four as you inhale.

4. Exhale slowly through your mouth: As you exhale, gently contract your belly, and release the air from your lungs. Count to four as you exhale.

5. Repeat the inhale and exhale cycle: Continue taking slow, deep breaths. Place your hands on your belly to feel your breath motions and concentrate on it.

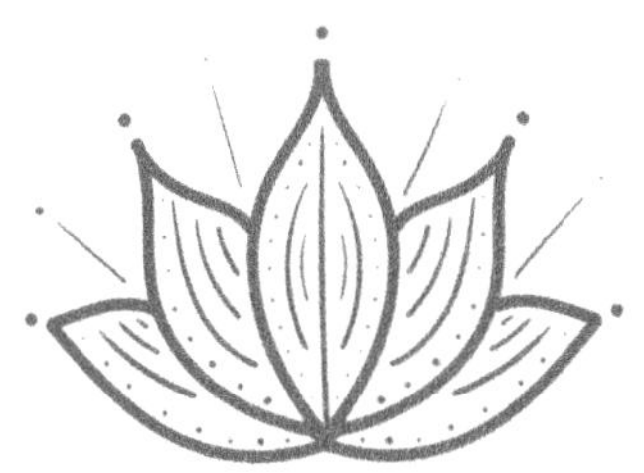

The Anjali Mudra, a fundamental pose in yoga, is often used at the beginning or end of a routine to center and focus the mind. In our 5-Step Chair Yoga Routine, we incorporate this pose as part of Step 2. While in Anjali Mudra, we will take the opportunity to set our Practice Intention.

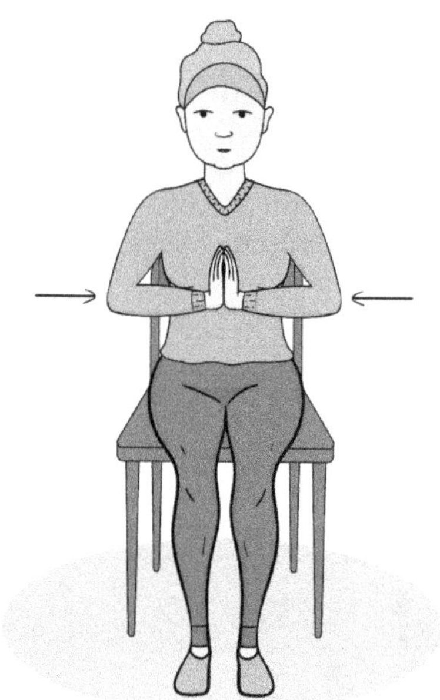

Limitations:

Easily accessible for seniors and individuals with mobility issues who may have difficulty getting down to and back up from the floor.

Benefits:

Easily accessible for seniors and individuals with mobility issues who may have difficulty getting down to and back up from the floor.

1. Sit on your chair, set your feet squarely on the ground and straighten your spine.

2. With your fingers pointing up, bring your palms together near your chest.

3. Press your palms together with gentle pressure.

4. Breathe using your nose with your eyes close

5. Remain in this position until you are ready to go on.

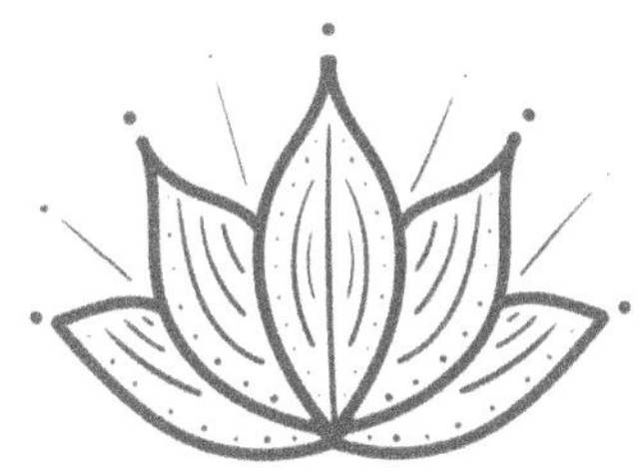

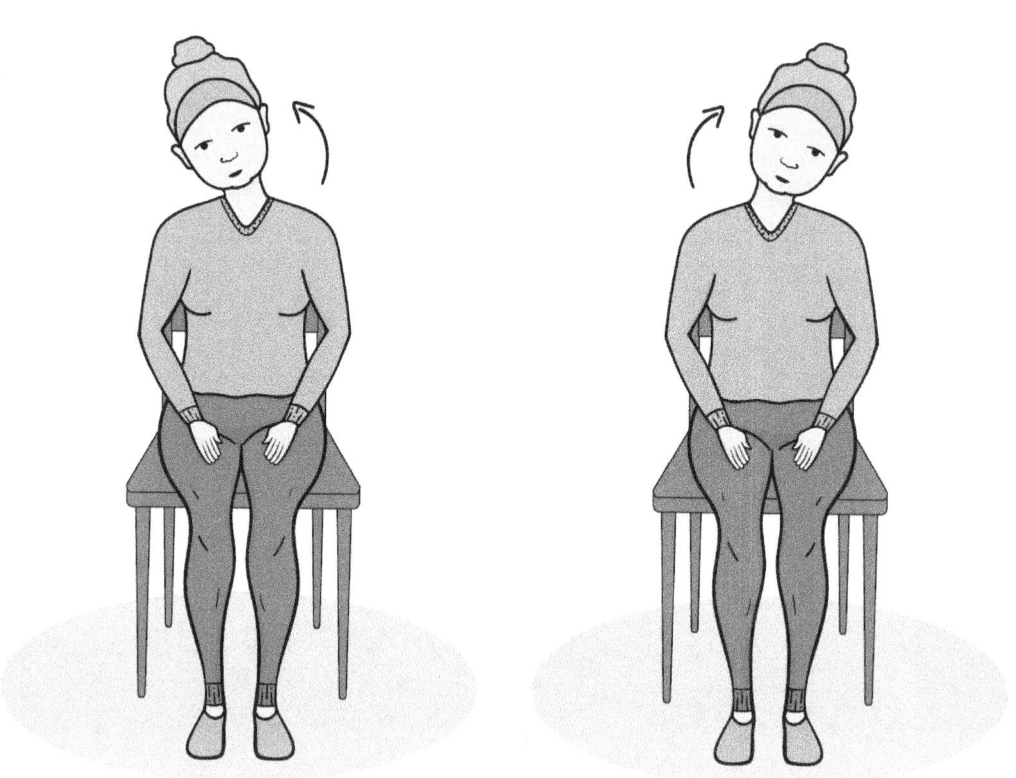

If you have neck injuries or have recently had neck surgery, avoid this pose. If you have limited neck mobility, be careful and perform the movements gently.

Benefits:

Relieves tension in the neck and shoulders, improves posture, enhances range of motion, and prevents injuries.

1. Sit on your chair, set your feet squarely on the ground and straighten your spine.
2. Inhale and move your head to bring your right ear to your right shoulder and hold.
3. Exhale and come back to Seated Basic Pose.
4. Repeat on the left side.
5. Come back to Seated Basic Pose.
6. Repeat.

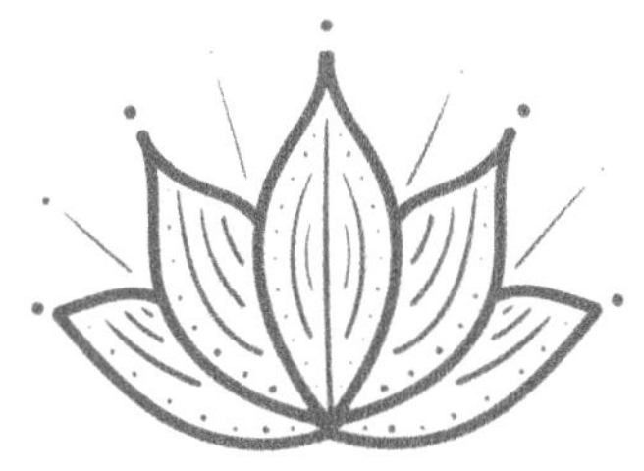

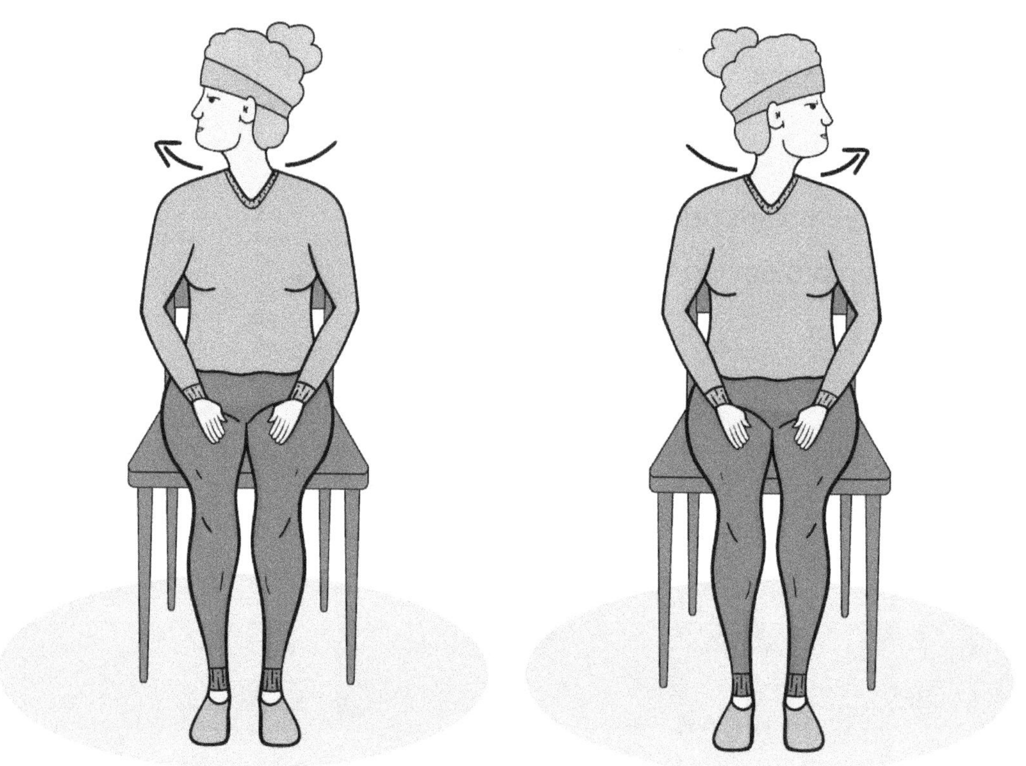

Limitations:

Avoid this pose if you have neck injuries or have recently undergone neck surgery. If you have limited neck mobility, be cautious and perform the movements gently.

Benefits:

This exercise helps relieve tension in the neck and shoulders, improves posture, enhances the range of motion, and can help prevent neck-related injuries.

1. Sit on your chair, straighten your spine, and place your feet firmly on the ground.

2. Gently move your neck in a circular motion, first taking your head up and then down, being careful not to strain.

3. Complete two rounds of this circular motion in one direction.

4. Then, gently repeat the circular motion in the opposite direction for another two rounds.

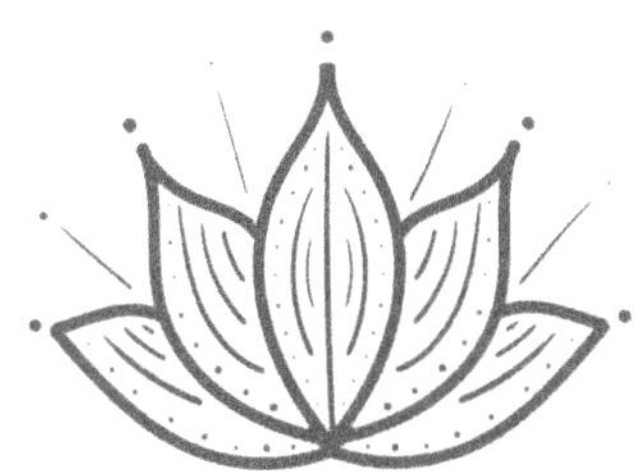

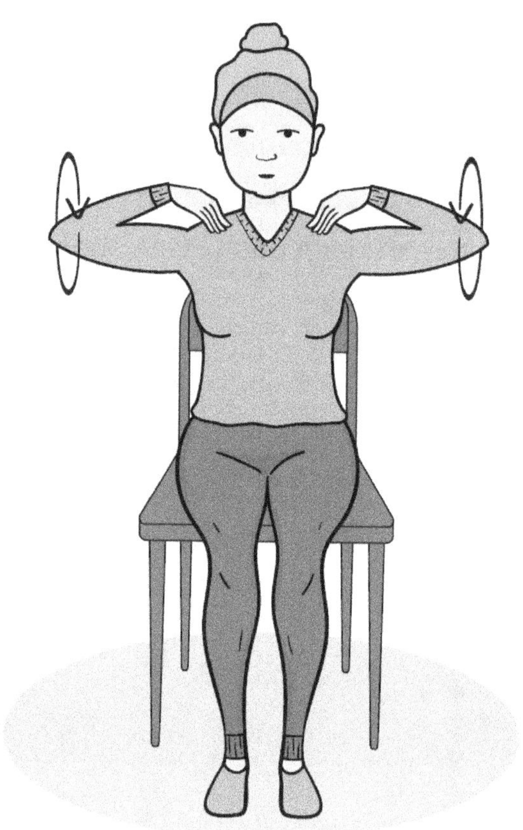

Limitations:

If you have shoulder injuries or conditions causing shoulder pain, perform this movement gently.

Benefits:

This exercise helps reduce stiffness and pain in the shoulders and improves circulation in the area.

1. Sit on your chair, set your feet squarely on the ground and straighten your spine.

2. Place your hands on your shoulders to guide the movement.

3. Gently roll your shoulders, lifting them up and then moving them back in a circular motion.

4. Perform four rounds of shoulder rolls in one direction.

5. Then, change direction and repeat the shoulder rolls for another four rounds in the opposite direction.

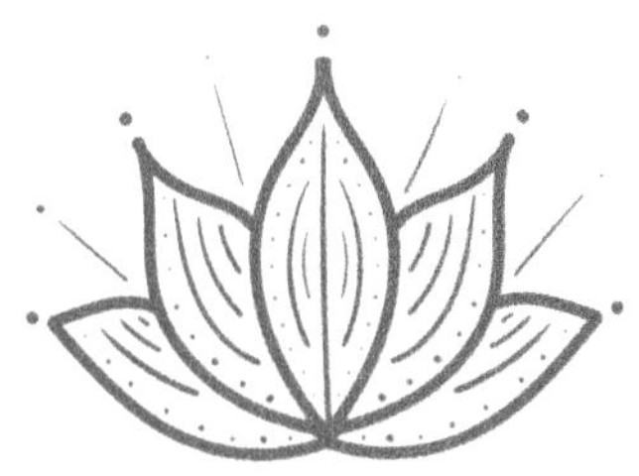

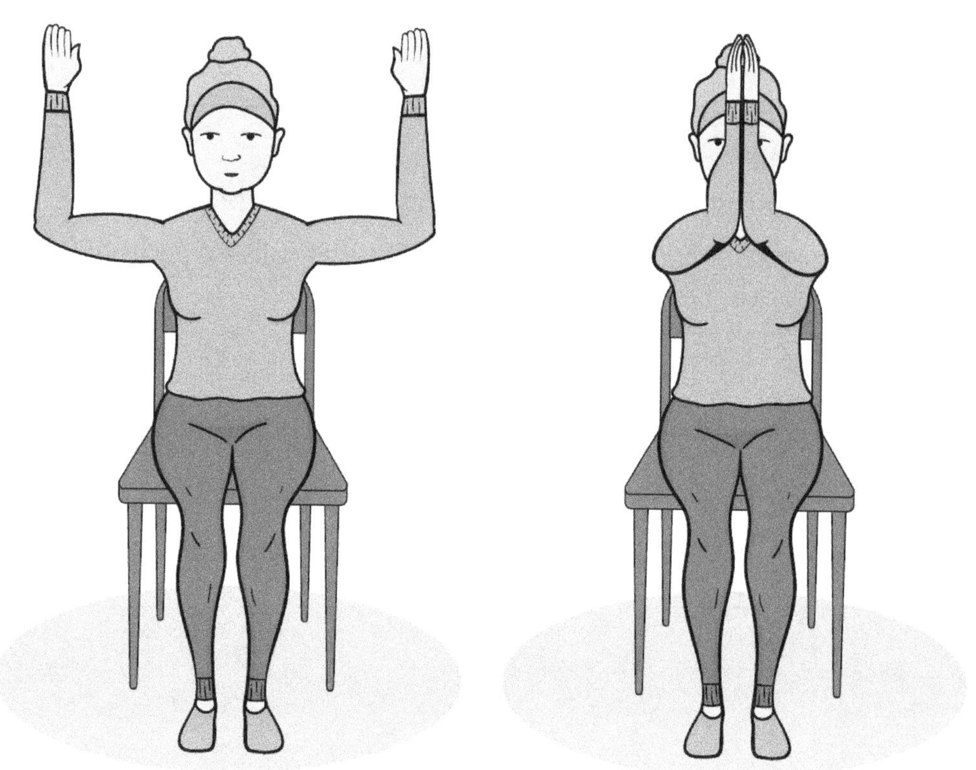

Limitations:

If you have shoulder conditions like frozen shoulders, avoid them.

Benefits:

Enhance your posture, upper back and shoulder mobility, and shoulder stress.

1. Sit on your chair, set your feet squarely on the ground and straighten your spine.

2. Bring your arms up to shoulder height, bending your elbows so that your finger points toward the ceiling.

3. Inhale and draw your elbows back, bringing your shoulder blades as close as you can.

4. Exhale and release, bringing your arms in front of you.

5. Repeat the movement, inhaling to draw the elbows back and exhaling to release them forward.

6. When you're ready to release the pose, inhale and bring your hands to your thighs.

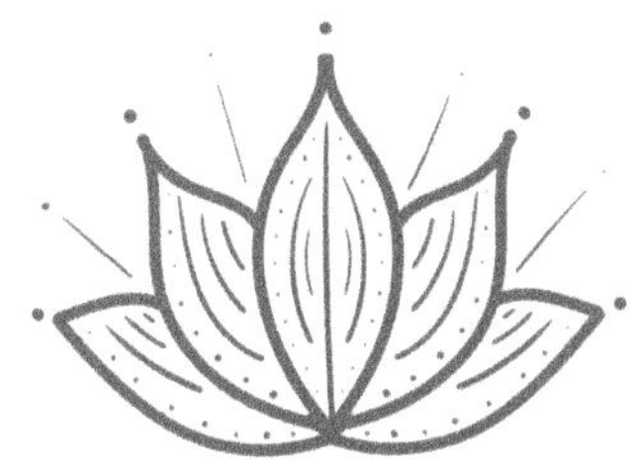

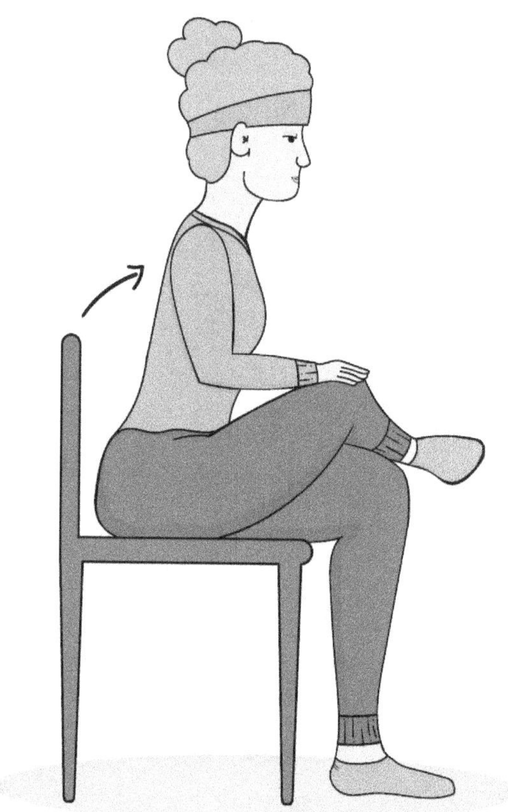

It can be challenging for people with knee or hip injuries or limited flexibility or mobility in the lower body.

Stretches quadriceps, improves balance, and engages core muscles.

1. Sit on your chair, straighten your spine, and place your feet firmly on the ground.
2. Bring your right ankle over your left thigh.
3. Inhale and stretch your spine up.
4. Exhale and move your back slightly forward, keeping it straight.
5. Hold for 3 breaths and slowly release.
6. Switch leg and repeat.

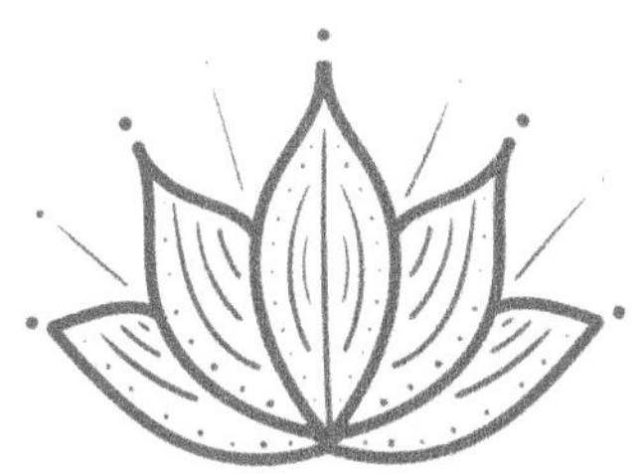

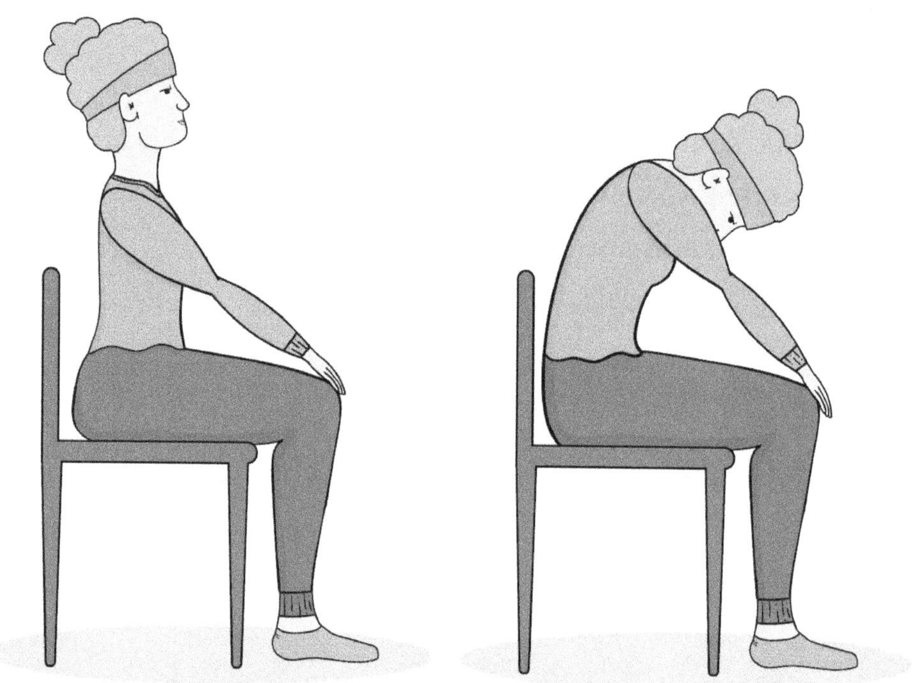

Limitations:

Be gentle or perform a variation if you have limited spinal mobility.

Benefits:

Releases tension in the spine, improves posture, massages internal organs, and promotes relaxation.

1. Sit on your chair, set your feet squarely on the ground and straighten your spine.

2. Inhale as you arch your spine back, bringing your shoulder blades together.

3. Then, round your spine and lower your chin toward your chest as you exhale.

4. Repeat 4 times.

8B Variation for limited spinal mobility people.

If you are not able to arc and round your back fully, try moving your pelvis forward and backward while keeping the spine almost straight.

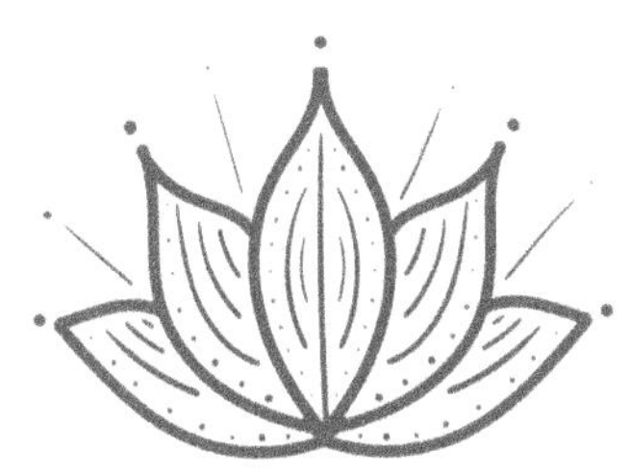

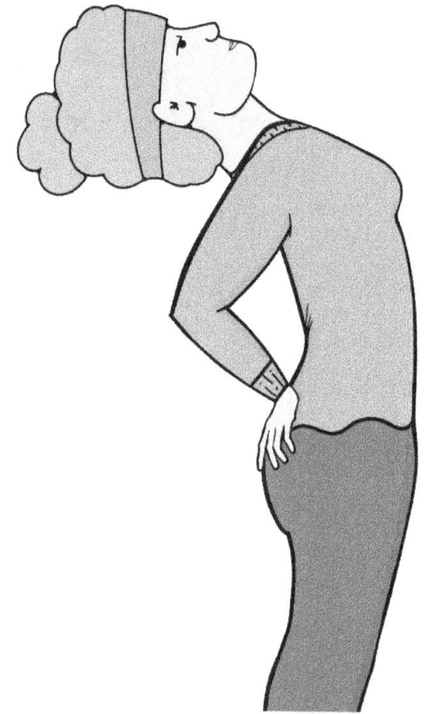

Limitations:

You need to be careful if you have herniated discs or back injuries. If you experience pain while performing the pose, pay attention to your body and stop.

Benefits:

Stretches the chest and shoulder, opens up the front body, improves posture, relieves tension in the back and neck, and stimulates organs in the abdomen.

1. Stand next to your chair, with your feet squarely on the ground and straighten your spine.
2. Inhale and bring your right hand to the base of your back.
3. Exhale and gently press your back forward with your hand while you rise.
4. Repeat, switching to the opposite side.

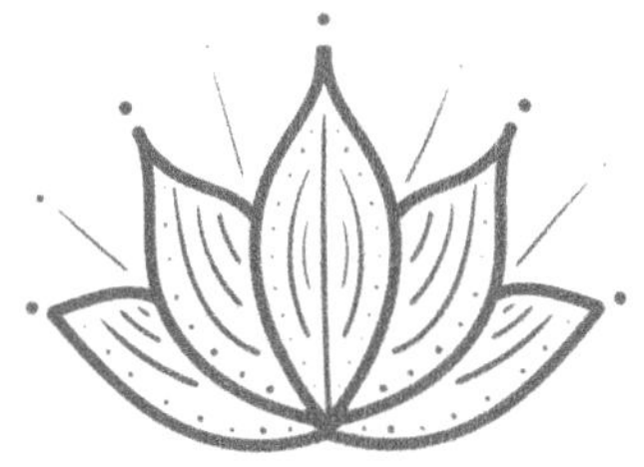

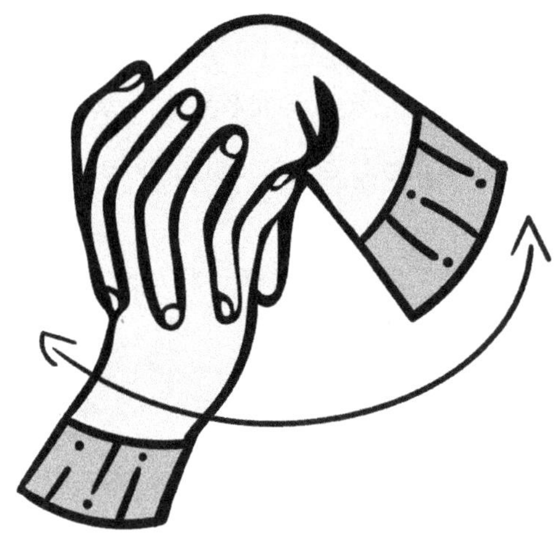

Limitations:

Avoid it if you suffer from Carpal Tunnel or Arthritis

Benefits:

Improves flexibility and range of motion in the wrist and hands, relieves tension, and can help to prevent wrist and hand injuries.

1. Sit on your chair, straighten your spine, and place your feet firmly on the ground.

2. Bring your palms together near your chest.

3. Interlock your fingers with your hands pointing up.

4. Slowly start to circle your hands and wrists clockwise, making small circles at first and gradually getting larger.

5. After 4 rotations, switch to a counterclockwise direction and repeat.

6. Continue circling for several rounds, breathing deeply and mindfully.

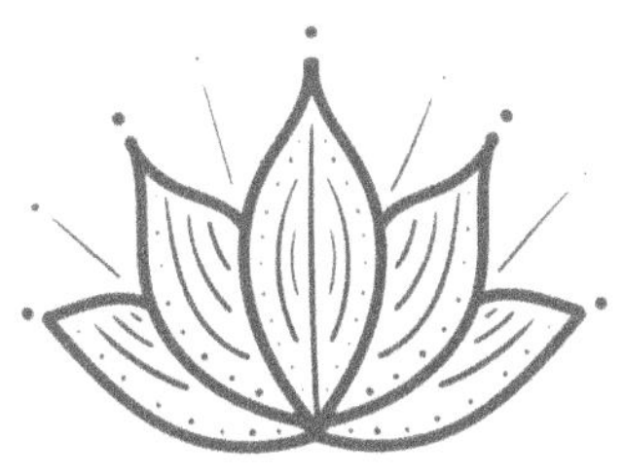

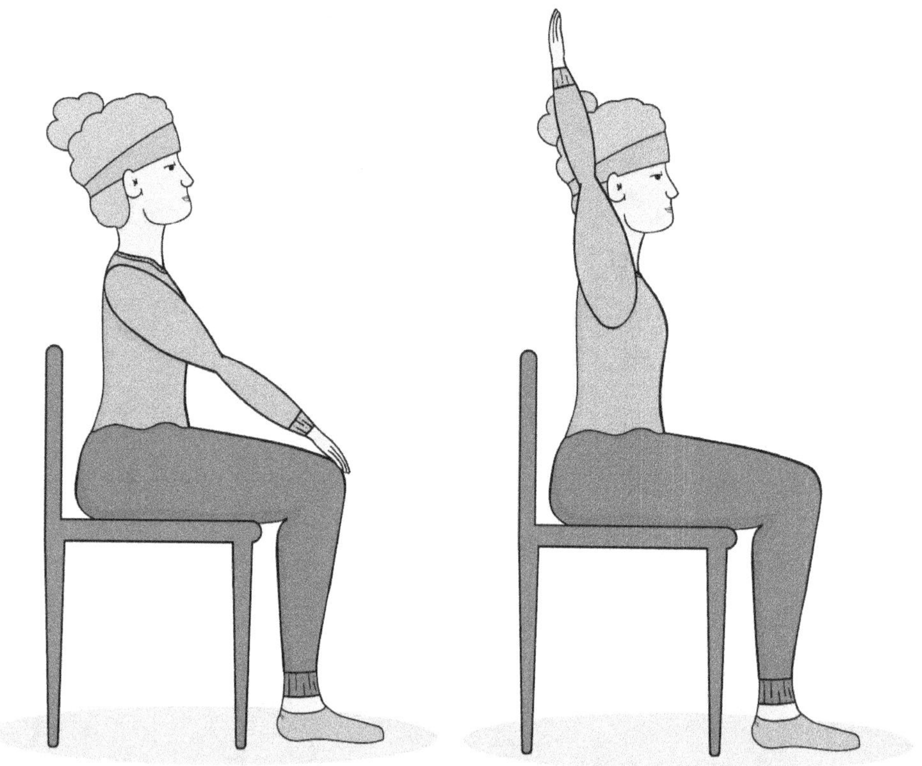

Avoid it if you have severed spine or back problems.

Improves posture, increases spine hip flexibility, helps to improve balance and stability, relieves tension in the shoulder and neck, and improves overall body awareness.

1. Sit on your chair, straighten your spine, and place your feet firmly on the ground.
2. Inhale and raise your arms.
3. Exhale and return your arms to their original position.
4. Repeat 4 times.

11B Variation for Dynamism

Introduce a variation by lowering your arms in 2 steps:

<u>First step:</u> Exhale halfway and bring your arms parallel to the ground, holding counting to 3.

<u>Second step:</u> Continue exhaling and bring your arms down.

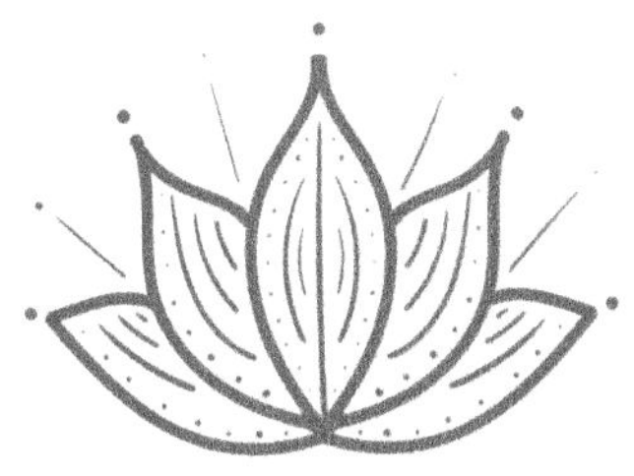

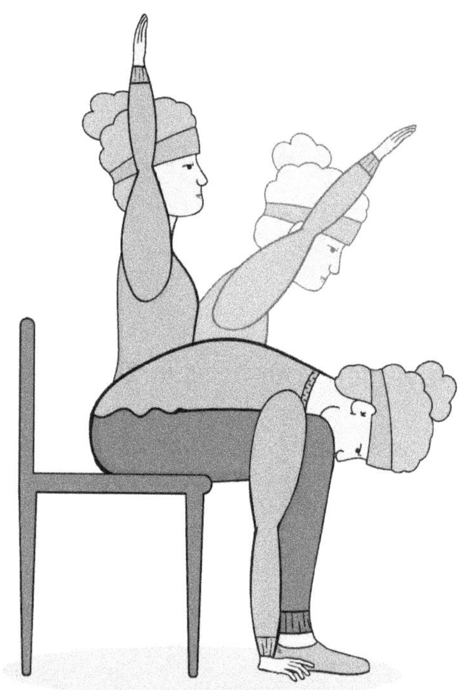

Perform carefully if you suffer from lower back pain and introduce the next variation if you have weak bones or osteoporosis to avoid round the spine.

Stretches the hamstrings, back, and neck muscles promote relaxation and relieve stress.

1. Sit on your chair, set your feet squarely on the ground and straighten your spine.
2. Inhale as you raise your arms in the air over your head.
3. As you exhale, bend over, and touch your toes.
4. Hold for 3 breaths, then come back up to seated.
5. Repeat 4 times.

128. Variation for People with Low Mobility, Flexibility, And Pain

Bend as much as you can but maintain your spine straight by bringing your chest up.

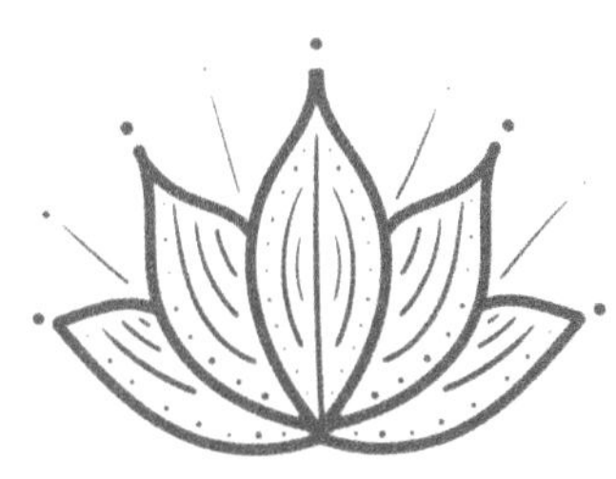

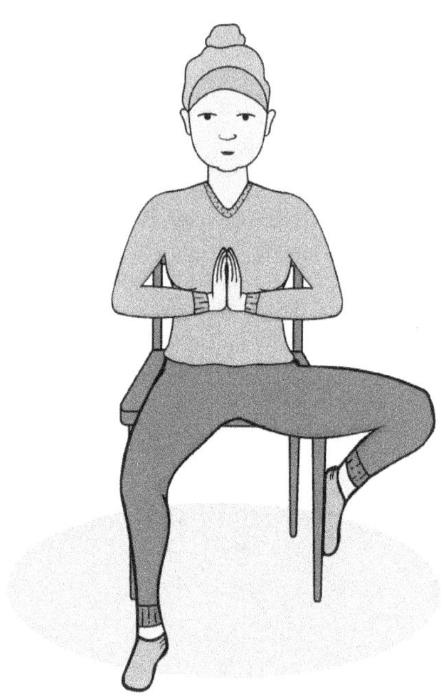

Limitations:

Perform carefully if you have limited motion in your hips or knees.

Benefits:

Strengthens the leg muscles, improves ankle stability, and can help to improve posture and balance, concentration, and focus.

1. Sit on your chair, straighten your spine, and place your feet firmly on the ground.
2. Transfer your weight to your right foot while raising your left foot off the ground.
3. Make sure your left knee is pointing outwards while placing the sole of your left foot on the front left leg of the chair.
4. Focusing on a fixed point in front of you, brings your hands together in front of your heart.
5. As you inhale, lengthen your spine, imagining your head reaching the ceiling.
6. As you exhale, press the leg of the chair with your right sole.
7. Hold the pose for a few breaths, feeling the strength in your legs and the sense of grounding through your feet.
8. To release, slowly lower your foot back to the ground and repeat on the opposite side by lifting your left foot and bringing it to your right thigh.

13B. Variation for more advanced people.

If you can, place the sole of your foot on the other leg, calf or tight. Always listen to your body.

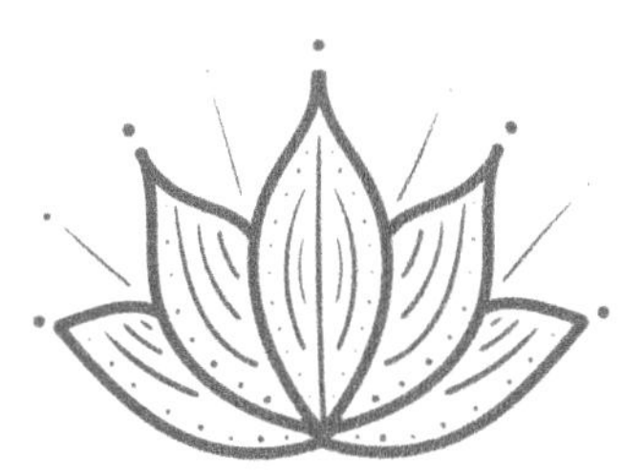

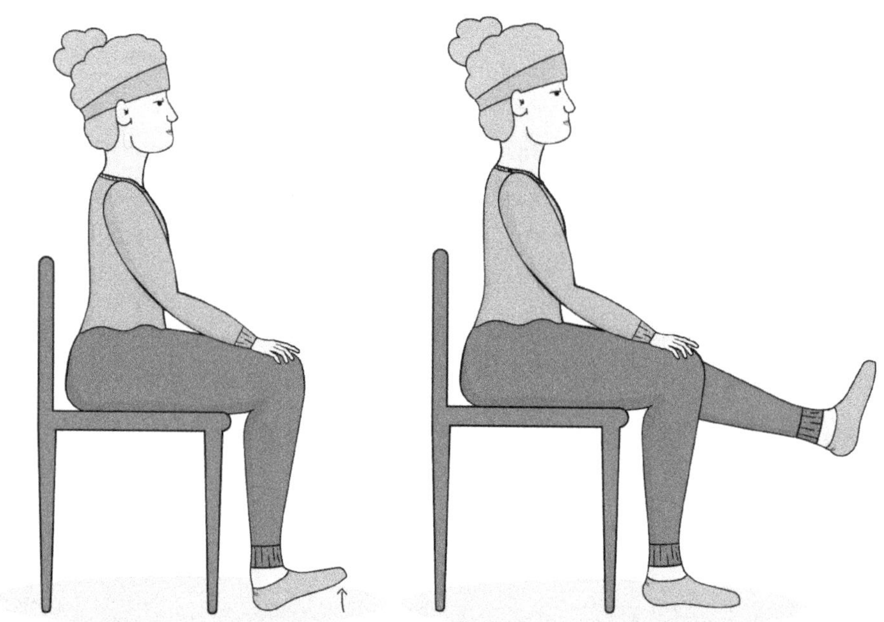

Limitations:

Perform with care if you have injuries in your foot or ankle.

Benefits:

Strengthens muscles of the feet and toes, improving balance and stability. Promotes foot flexibility.

1. Sit on your chair, straighten your spine, and place your feet firmly on the ground.
2. Inhale and lift the toes off the ground, keeping the heels of the feet grounded.
3. Exhale and lift your heels off the ground, keeping your toes grounded.
4. Repeat 4 times.
5. Then, raise your foot off the floor while transferring your weight to the other, and hold for 4 seconds.
6. Turn back the Seated Base Position and Tap your toes on the ground.
7. Using the left and right feet alternately.
8. Repeat 5 times.

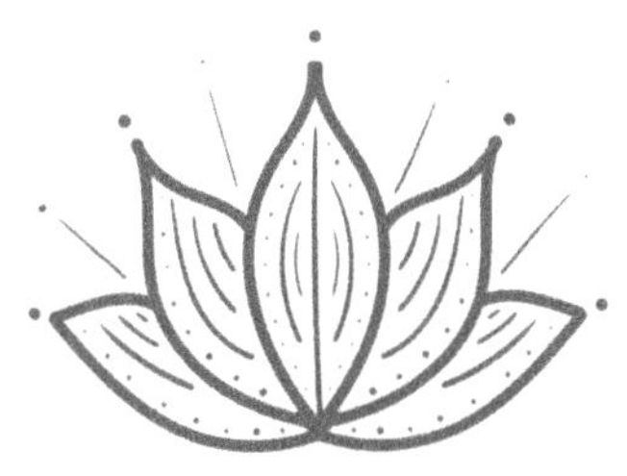

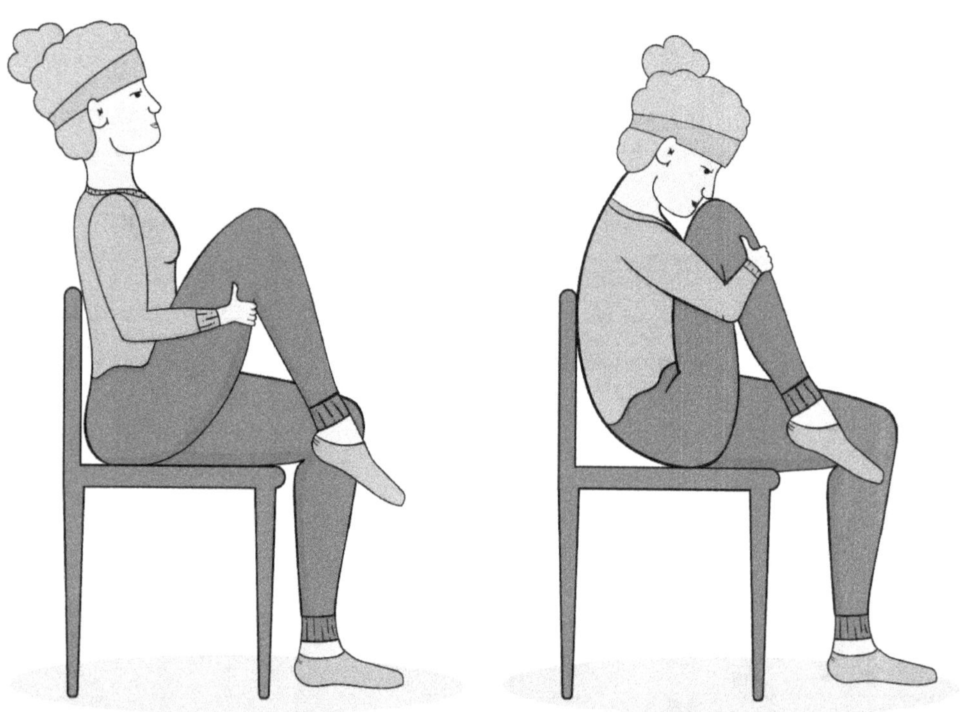

Pay special attention if you have hips and knee mobility limitations.

Release tension in the hips and lower back.

1. Sit on your chair, straighten your spine, and place your feet firmly on the ground.

2. Bring one knee up to your chest and grab it with both hands.

3. Bring it gently close to your chest. Notice the stretch in your hip and lower back.

4. Keep the other foot on the ground.

5. Hold the pose for 3 breaths, then release and switch sides.

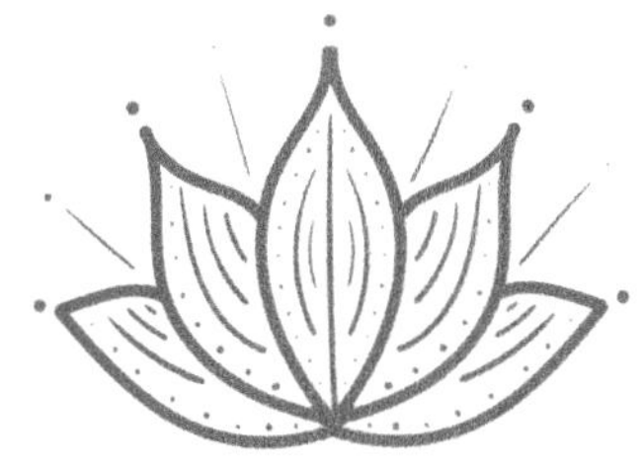

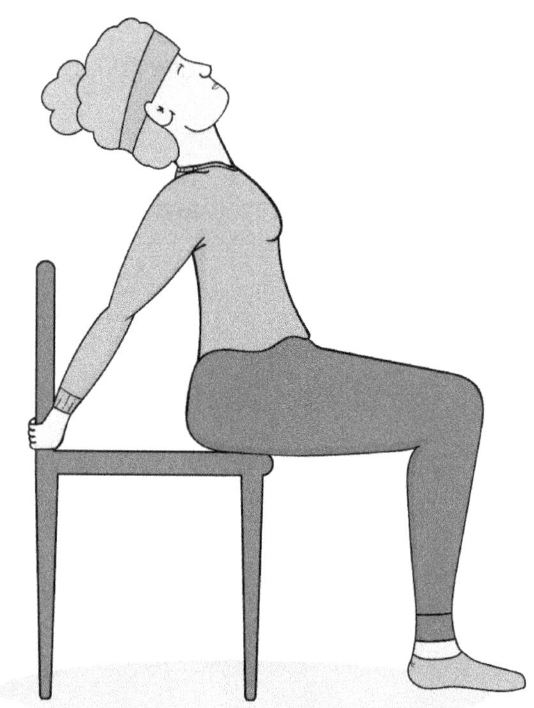

People with recent abdominal or back surgery should avoid this pose.

Improve circulation, flexibility, and balance.

Instructions:

1. Sit on your chair, set your feet squarely on the ground and straighten your spine.

2. Inhale and lift your chest up, arching your back and keeping your elbows close to your side.

3. Look up and breathe deeply.

4. Hold the pose for 3 breaths, then release.

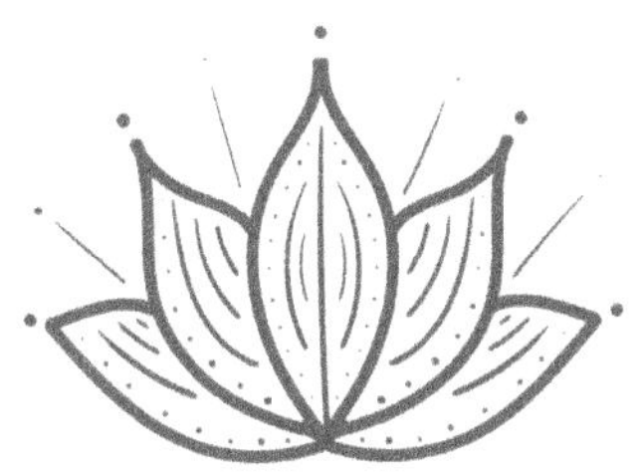

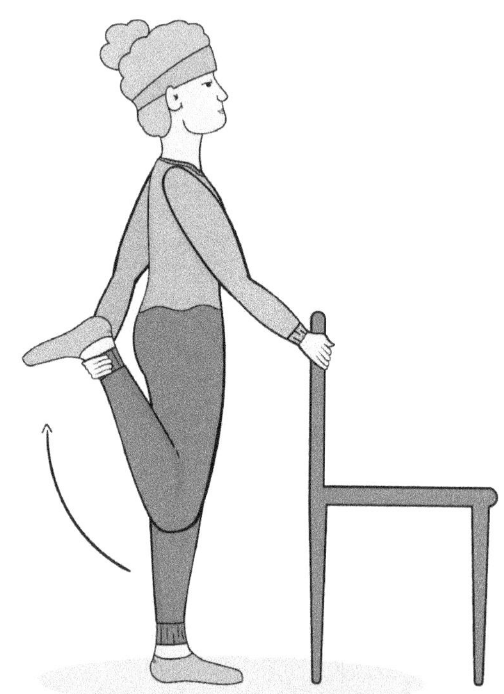

If you have balance issues, make sure to use a stable chair for support. If you suffer from tight quadriceps, you may need to introduce a variation.

Improves flexibility and balance and reduces the risk of injury.

Instructions:

1. Stand behind the chair with your feet hip-width apart.
2. Use your left hand to hold onto the chair's back and bend your right knee, bringing your heel toward your buttocks.
3. Use your right hand to hold your ankle or foot as you feel a stretch in the front of your right thigh.
4. Keep your left leg straight and engage your core to maintain balance.
5. Hold for 3 breaths, then release and switch sides.

17B Variations for People with Tight Quadriceps:

If your quadriceps are tight, you may not be able to reach your ankle or foot. In this case, you can use a strap or towel to help you hold onto your foot or simply reach

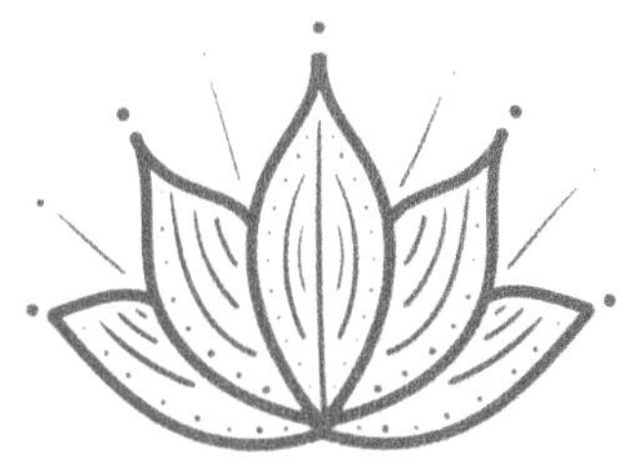

back as far as you can without straining. Be careful with your balance.

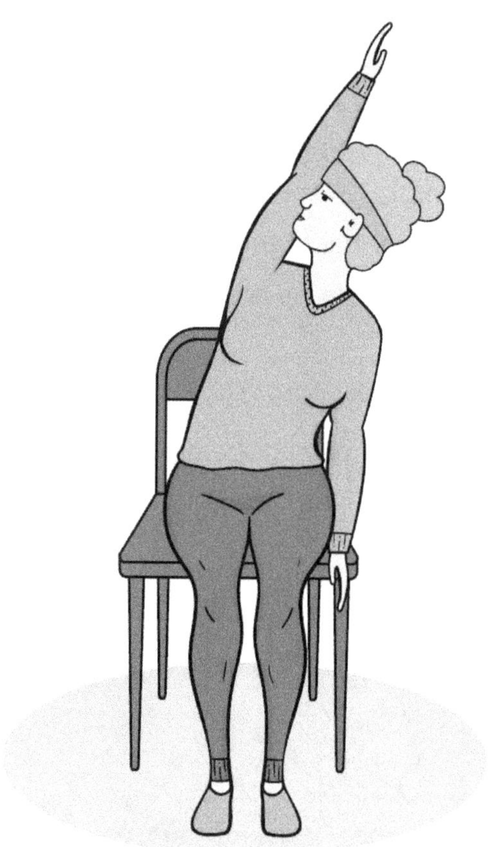

If you have spinal issues perform this pose carefully.

Increase range of motion.

Instructions:

1. Sit on your chair, straighten your spine, and place your feet firmly on the ground.
2. Reach one arm up towards the ceiling.
3. Inhale and lengthen the spine.
4. As you exhale, gently side bend towards the opposite side, taking care not to fall into the side of the chair.
5. Hold the stretch for 3 breaths and release.
6. Return to the center and repeat on the other side.

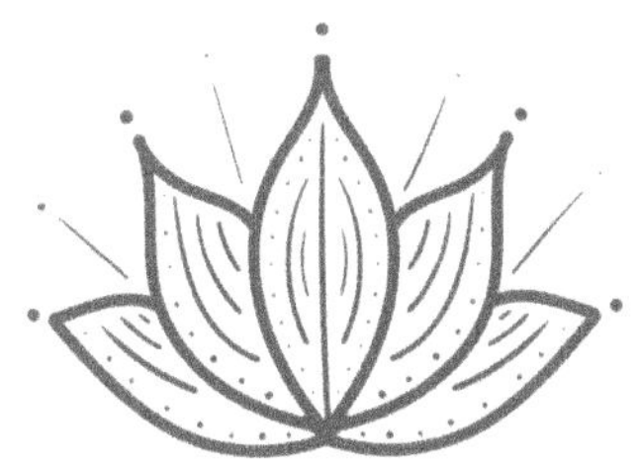

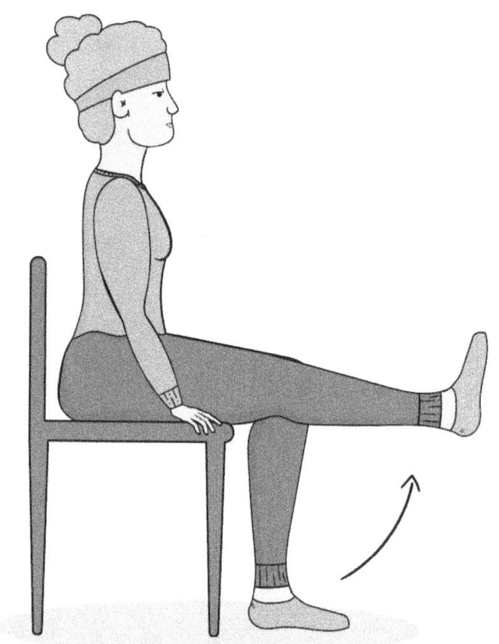

Limitations:

If you feel extreme pain in your knees or hamstring while doing the pose, stop it. People with hip pain may find it difficult to extend their legs fully.

Benefits:

Strengthens muscles of the feet and toes, improving balance and stability. Promotes foot flexibility.

Instructions:

1. Sit on your chair, set your feet squarely on the ground and straighten your spine.
2. Inhale and lift one of your legs, extending it out in front of you.
3. Exhale and lower your leg back down to the floor.
4. Repeat on the left side, then switch sides.
5. Continue alternating sides, focusing on deep breathing and engaging your core.

19B Variation for People with Lower Back Pain

If you have lower back pain, you may need to modify this pose by putting a folded blanket or cushion to support your back.

19C Variation for People with Flexibility Limitations

If you can't fully extend your leg, don't force it extend it as far as you can. You will experience increased flexibility over time.

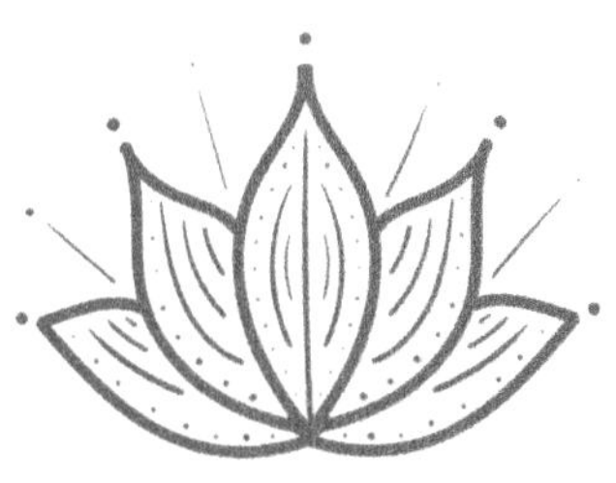

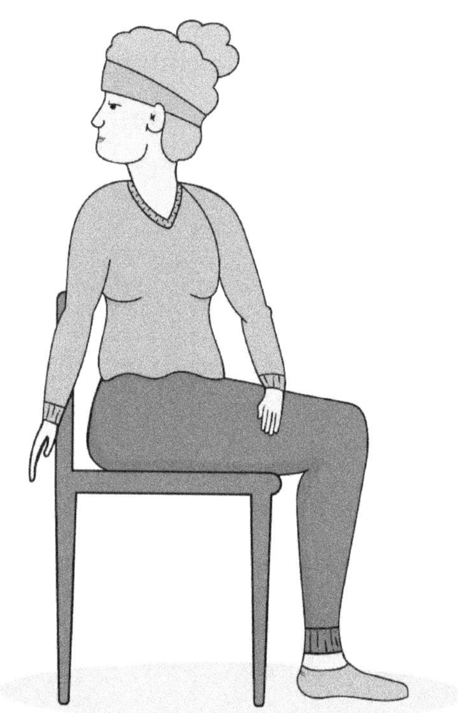

Limitations:

If you have back pain or a herniated disk, avoid or practice with precaution.

Benefits:

Improves spinal mobility, stretches the spine, shoulders, and neck, and stimulates digestion.

1. Sit on your chair, set your feet squarely on the ground and straighten your spine.

2. Inhale and lengthen the spine.

3. Exhale and rotate your upper body to the right, directing your movement by bringing your left hand to your right knee.

4. Hold for 2 to 5 breaths, then come back to the center.

5. Repeat on the left side.

6. Continue alternating sides for two minutes, concentrate on inhaling deeply and contracting your abs.

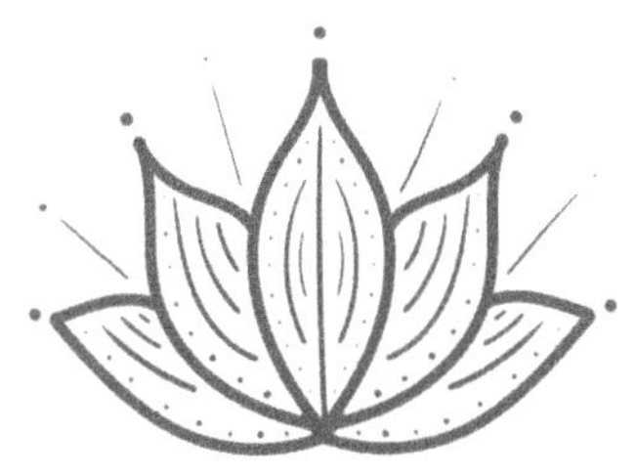

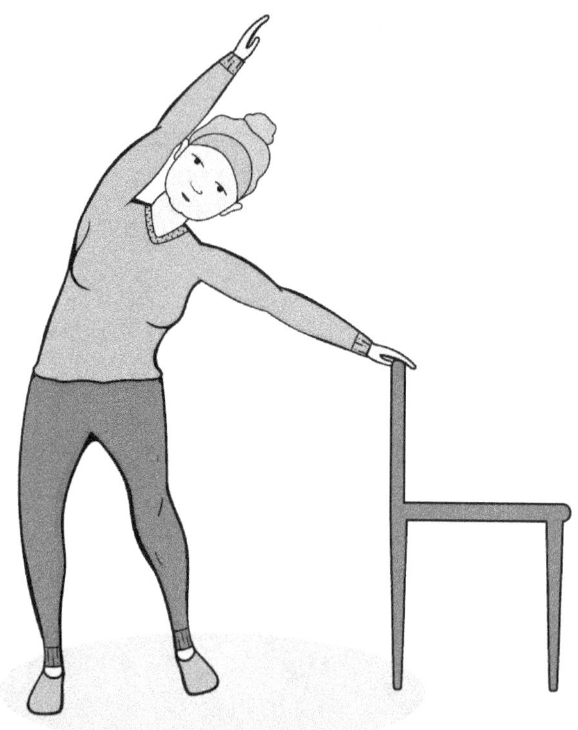

Be careful if you have neck, spine, or back pain. Standing side stretches can be difficult for people with balance issues and cause dizziness.

Benefits:

Stretches the entire side of the body.

1. Stand facing the chair with your feet hip-width apart.

2. Take a deep breath and raise your right arm upwards while holding onto the chair's back with your left hand.

3. Exhale as you stretch your right arm to the left, feeling a gentle stretch down the right side of your body.

4. Hold for 3 breaths before switching sides.

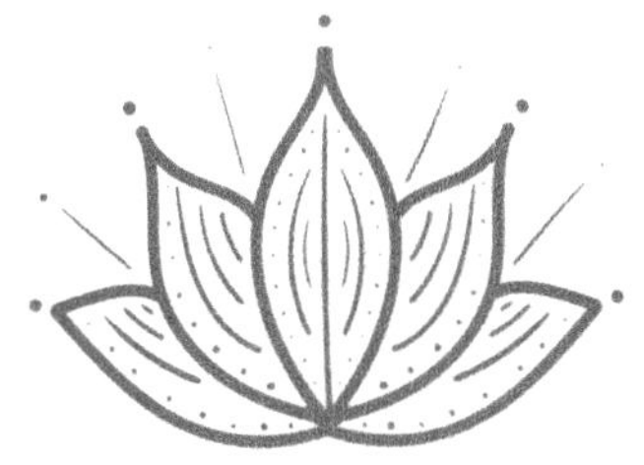

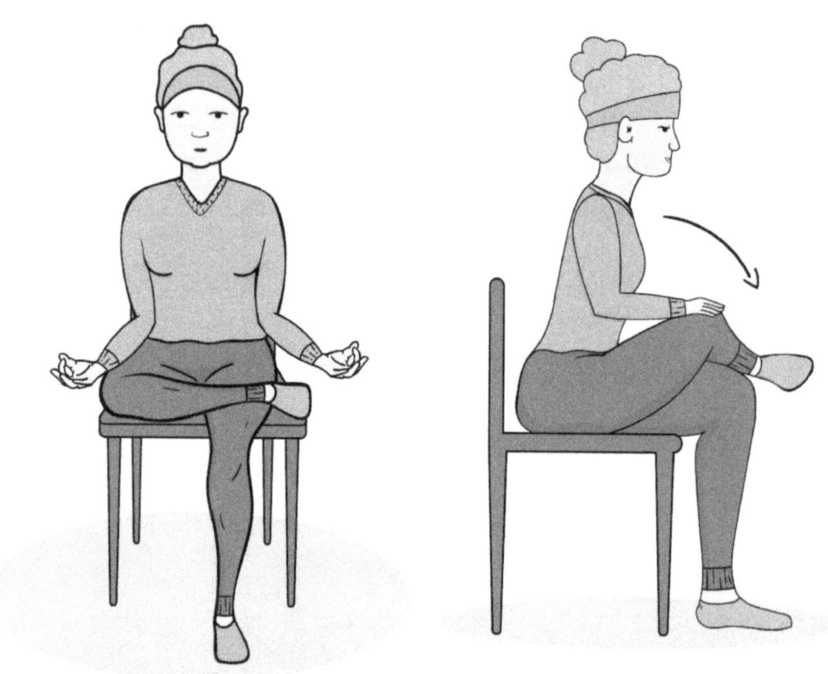

Limitations:

If you have knee or ankle injuries, avoid this pose. If you experience any pain or discomfort, come out of the pose.

Benefits:

Increase hip flexibility, alleviate tightness in the hips and lower back, and can improve overall posture.

1. Sit on your chair, straighten your spine, and place your feet firmly on the ground.

2. Rest your right ankle on your left knee while letting your right knee slouch slightly to the side.

3. While maintaining a straight back, arch forward at the hips to move your chest toward your right knee.

4. With your hands on your right knee, gently press down while noticing how your hip is being stretched.

5. Hold the pose, then release and switch sides.

22B Variation for People Interested in Losing Weight

For a more dynamic version, try moving in and out of the pose with each exhale and inhale.

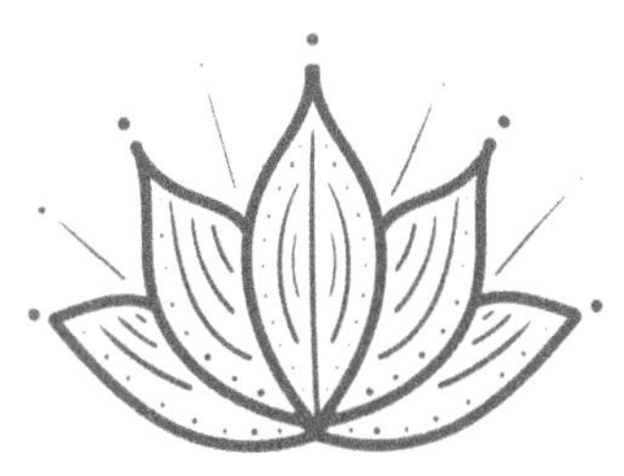

More Challenging Poses (Intermediate-Advance)

These poses require a bit more strength, balance, and flexibility and may include variations of the basic poses, as well as new poses that challenge the body and mind.

23A Chair Pose (Utkatasana)

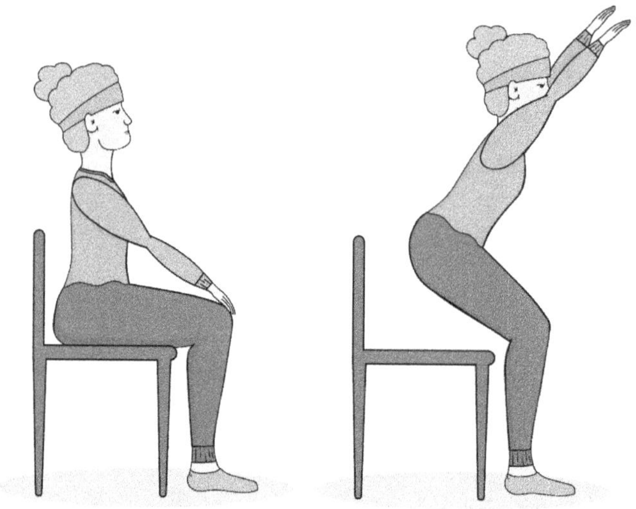

Limitations:

If you suffer from knee pain, you may find it uncomfortable to hold the pose for an extended period. If you suffer from low back pain or severe balance issue you may need to introduce a variation

Benefits:

Strengthening the legs and core, improving balance, and increasing endurance

1. Sit on your chair, straighten your spine, and place your feet hip-width apart firmly on the ground.

2. Lift your arms upward.

3. As you inhale, get up from your chair, lift your chest and bring your shoulders down and back.

4. As you exhale, bend your knees, and lower your hips toward the chair as if you are about to sit down.

5. Keep your weight properly distributed between both feet and your knees in line with your ankles.

6. Maintain the position for 4 breaths, then inhale and straighten your legs to release.

23B Variation for People with Back Pain

If you suffer from low back pain or injury, you can modify the pose by placing your hands on your hips, instead of raising them.

23C Variation for People with Severe Balance Issues

If you suffer from severe balance issues, bend just slightly your knees and place your hands on your thighs instead of raising them.

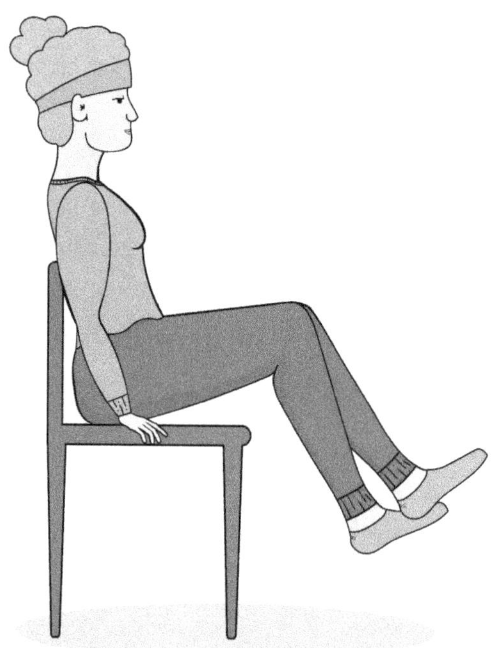

If you suffer from back, hip, or knee pain, pay special attention, it can be difficult to perform this pose. Consider that it is important to keep the back straight, avoiding rounding the spine.

Improves core strength and stability.

1. Sit on your chair, straighten your spine, and place your feet hip-width apart firmly on the ground.
2. Inhale and lift your feet slowly off the ground while maintaining your knees bent by contracting your abdominal muscles. Exhale while maintaining the position.
3. If necessary, hold on to the chair's sides for balance.
4. Inhale and get your legs straight with your toes pointing upward.
5. Maintain the position while extending your spine and lifting your chest upward.
6. Repeat 4 times, one complete breathing cycle for each part of the pose.
7. Gently bring your feet back to the floor.

24B Variation for people with limited mobility

If you have mobility or flexibility issues, you may find it difficult to maintain the proper form in a seated boat pose. Use a cushion in your lower back to make the pose more accessible.

24C Variation for people with balance issues.

If it is difficult for you to maintain this pose, you can place a block or another chair in front of you as a base. When you get tired or about to lose your balance, use it as a base to rest your feet in a higher position.

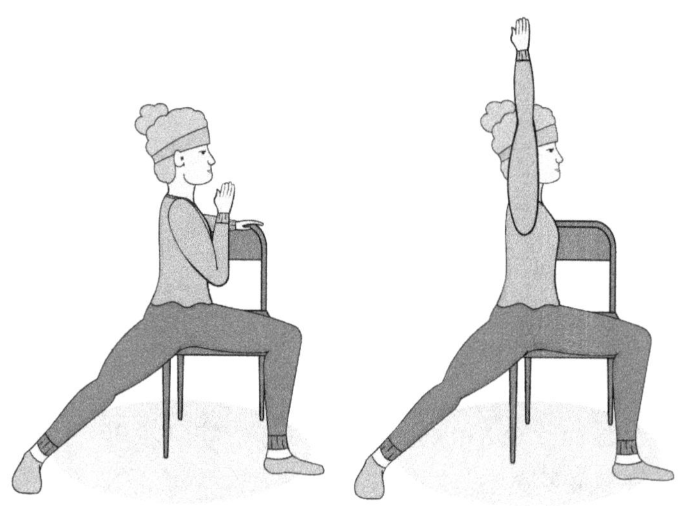

Limitations:

If you suffer from knee and hip pain or balance issues, you may need to modify this pose.

Benefits:

Strengthen and stretch the ankles, legs, shoulders, and arms.

Instructions:

1. To start, place yourself on one side of the chair with feet hip-width apart.
2. With your toes pointing forward, step your left foot forward and place it on the other side of the chair.
3. Bend your left knee, bringing it to a 90-degree angle and making sure it is directly above your left ankle.

4. Verify that your thigh is parallel to the ground and that your knee is squarely above your ankle.

5. Breathe in while raising your arms upward, with your palms together.

6. If you can, look up towards your hands, keeping your gaze forward and steady.

7. Hold the pose for 5 deep breaths. Focus on your balance and stability.

8. Release the pose, lowering your hands to your hips and straightening your left leg.

9. Repeat with the other leg.

25B Variation for People with Balance Issues

If it is difficult to raise the arms overhead, the hands can be placed on the hips or the chair for support.

25C Variation for People with Knee and Hip Pain

If it is difficult to perform this pose, you can stay seated and do just the upper body movements.

25D Variation for People Who Want to Strengthen Muscles and Lose Weight.

For a more advanced and active variation, perform this position outside the chair, lifting your back leg off the floor, maintaining it straight, and bringing the foot to the seat of the chair.

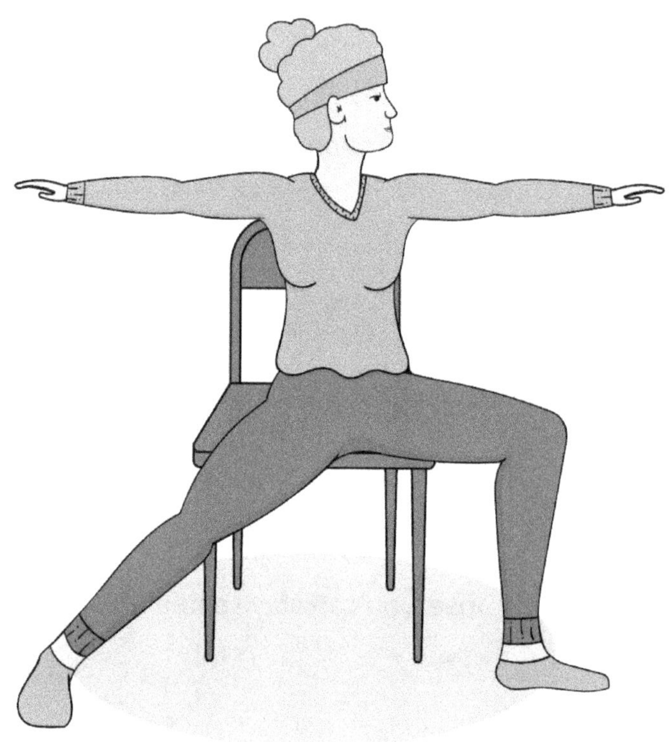

If you suffer from knee and hip pain, modify this pose.

Strengthens and stretches the legs and hips, while improving balance and stability

1. Sit on your chair, straighten your spine, and place your feet hip-width apart firmly on the ground and fingers softened and rest on your knees.

2. Extend your right leg behind you, keeping it straight and strong.

3. Bend your left knee, bringing it to a 90-degree angle and making sure it is directly above your left ankle.

4. With your arms parallel to your shoulders, extend them out to the sides.

5. Gaze out over your left fingertips, engaging your core and keeping your hips facing forward.

6. Take a few deep breaths in this position, feeling the stretch in your hips and the opening through your chest.

7. To release, lower your arms and bring first your back foot to the original position.

8. Repeat on the other side.

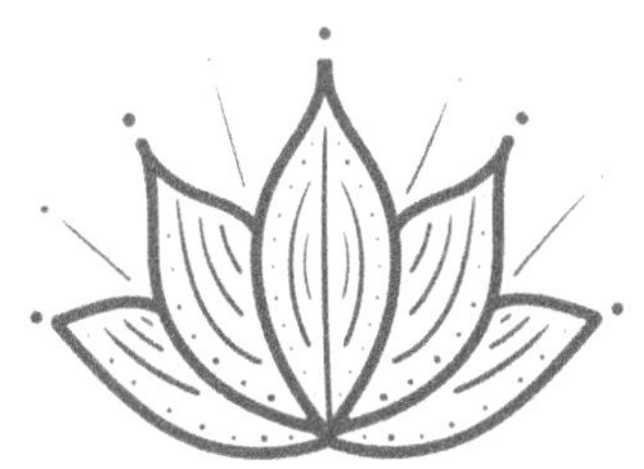

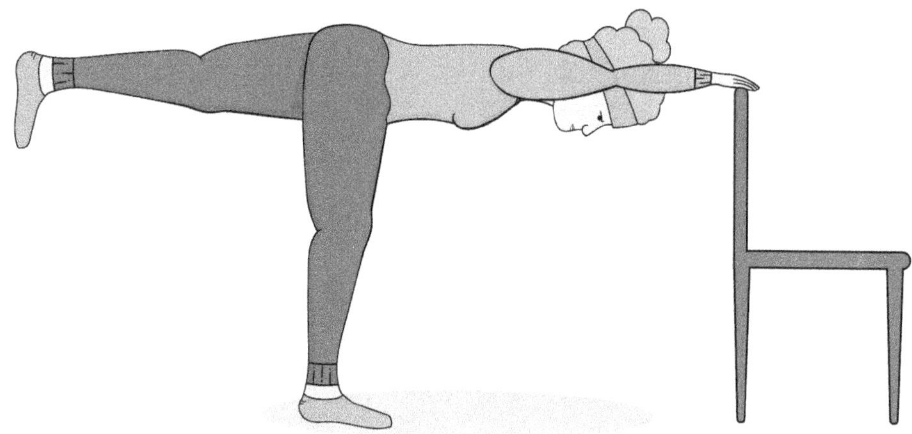

Limitations:

This pose requires balance, stability, and strength in the legs, core, and back muscles.

Benefits:

Improves balance, strengthens the lower body and core, and stretches hamstrings and back muscles.

1. To start, place yourself behind the chair with your feet aligned with your hip and your hands on the chair's top rail.

2. Transfer your weight to your left foot and extend your right leg behind you while lifting your right leg off the ground.

3. Reach your arms forward and engage your core as you hinge forward from the hips, bringing your torso parallel to the floor.

4. Keep your lifted leg aligned with your torso and reach your arms forward, lengthening through your fingertips.

5. Hold for a few breaths, then let go of the position and repeat on the other side.

27B Variation for People with Limited Flexibility

If you have flexibility issues, you may find it difficult to perform this pose. In this case, you can put your hands in the seat of the chair (instead of the top rail) and lift your leg off the ground, without bringing your torso parallel to the floor, but just tilting forward.

If the chair seat is very low, help yourself by putting a block over the seat to support your hands at a higher level and improve posture.

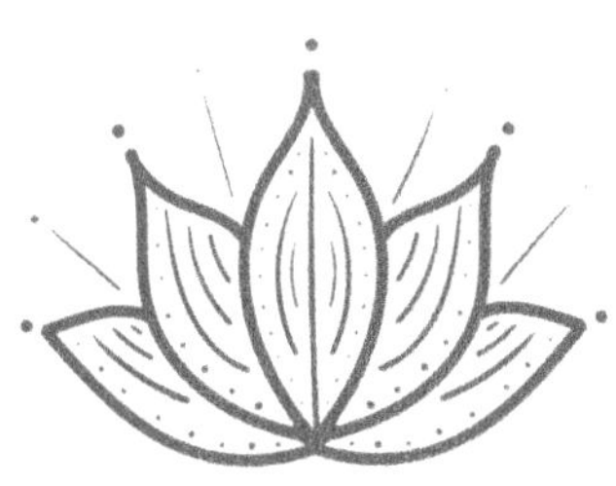

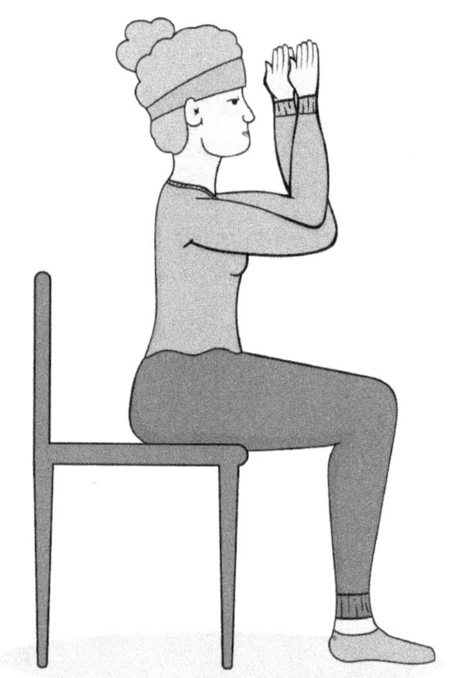

Limitations:

If you suffer from shoulder or elbow injuries, avoid this pose. If you have arthritis, you may find it challenging to bring your arms together and hold the pose for an extended period.

Benefits:

Reducing tension and stress in the upper body, improving posture and spinal alignment, and enhancing focus and concentration.

Instructions:

1. Sit on your chair, straighten your spine, and place your feet hip-width apart firmly on the ground and fingers softened and rest on your knees.

2. Bend your arms in front of you.

3. Inhale and take your right arm under your left, bringing your hands together and facing one another in front of your chest.

4. Staying in the pose, breathing deeply for a moment, and release.

5. Repeat on the opposite side.

28B Variation for People with Limited Flexibility

If you have flexibility issues, you may find it difficult to perform this pose. You can wrap one arm over the other as usual but bring your arms onto your shoulder instead of facing one another.

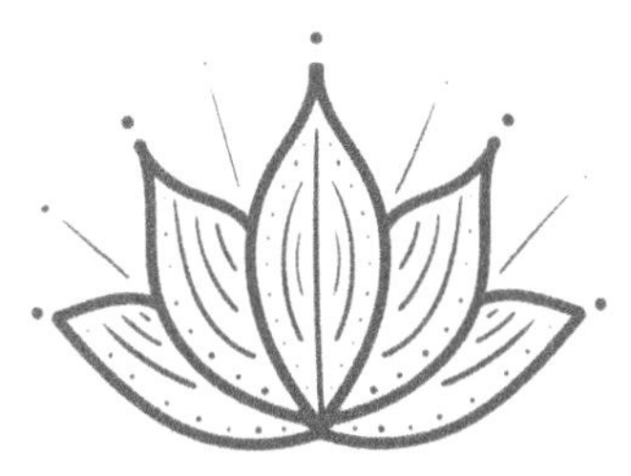

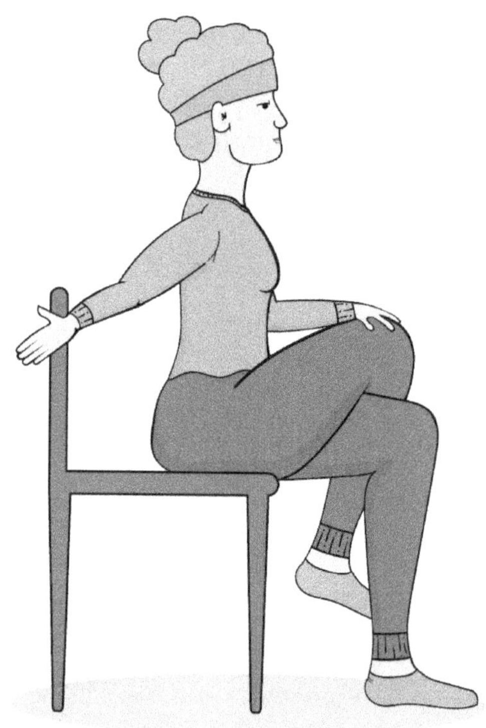

Limitations:

If you have hip or knee injuries may need to modify the pose or avoid it

Benefits:

Stretching the outer hip and thigh, improving balance and stability, and increasing focus and concentration

Instructions:

1. Sit on your chair, straighten your spine, and place your feet hip-width apart firmly on the ground and fingers softened and rest on your knees.
2. Cross your right leg over your left thigh.
3. Flex your right foot and put it behind your left calf.
4. Stay in the pose for 4 breaths, then release and switch sides.

29B Variation for People to Improve Balance.

To improve balance, while performing this pose, you can lengthen your spine by raising your arms aloft with your hands facing one another.

29C Variation for People to Improve Flexibility (Twisted Eagle Legs)

This variation adds a twist to the Chair Eagle Legs pose to improve flexibility. Bring your right hand to the chair's back and your left hand to your right knee while holding this position. Expand your spine as you inhale. Take a breath out, turn to the right, and glance over your right shoulder. After a few breaths of holding, release. Repeat, On the opposite side.

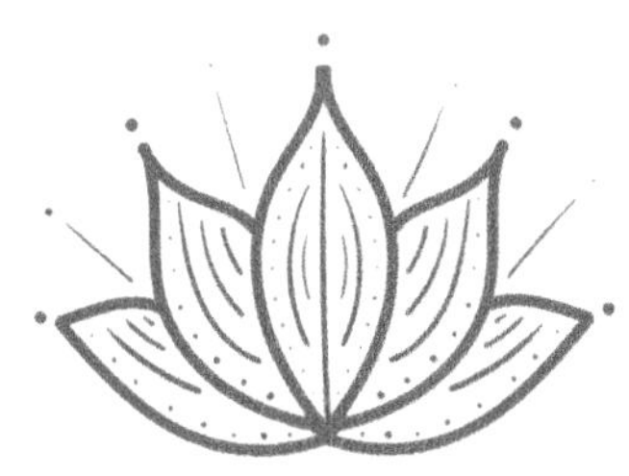

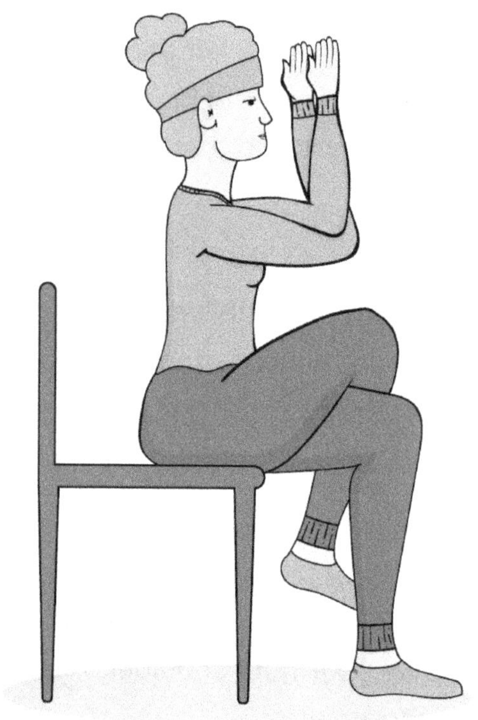

If you have hip or knee injuries may need to modify the pose or avoid it

Stretches shoulder and upper back, strengthens legs and hips, improves concentration and balance.

1. Sit on your chair, straighten your spine, and place your feet hip-width apart firmly on the ground and fingers softened and rest on your knees.

2. Cross your right thigh over your left and position your right foot behind the calf of your left leg.

3. For a deeper stretch, wrap your right foot behind your left calf.

4. Inhale and take your right arm under your left, bringing your hands together and facing one another in front of your chest.

5. Staying in the pose, breathing deeply for a moment, and then release.

6. Repeat on the opposite side.

30B Variation for People with Flexibility Issues

If you have difficulty bringing the leg over the opposite thigh, you can simply cross the ankles.

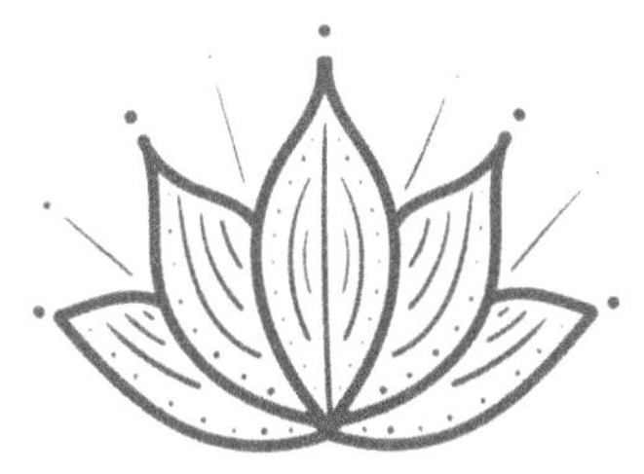

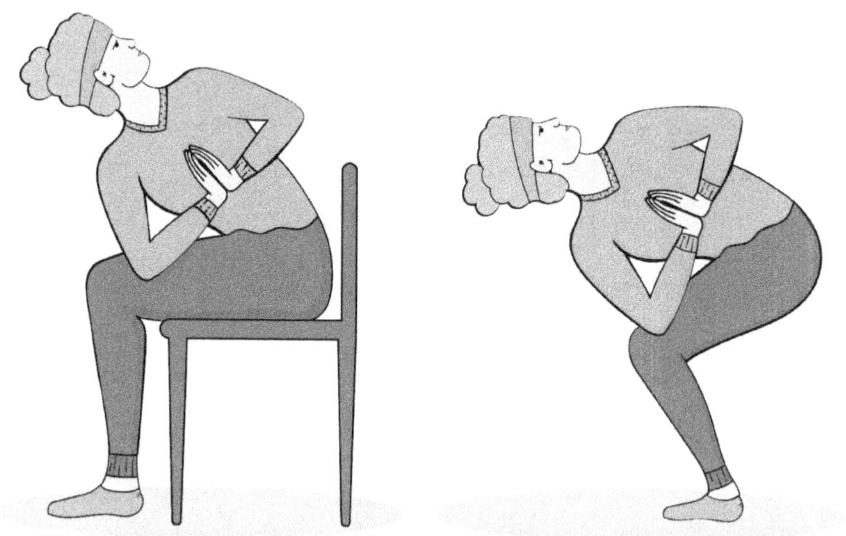

Limitations:

If you have hip problems such as hip arthritis or labral tear, avoid this pose.

Benefits:

Stretches arms and spine, improving balance and posture.

1. Sit on your chair, straighten your spine, and place your feet hip-width apart firmly on the ground and fingers softened and rest on your knees.

2. Take a deep breath in and lift your arms with your palms in a prayer pose.

3. Take a deep breath out while rotating your torso to the left and put your right elbow on the outside of your left knee.

4. Maintain this posture for a few breaths while feeling your hips, shoulders, and spine stretched.

5. Inhale and return to the center, lowering your arms.

6. Repeat switching sides.

31.B Variation for People to Improve Balance and Leg Strength.

Perform this pose, starting by standing up in front of the chair and bending your knees as if you are sitting on the chair. Then continue with standard instructions.

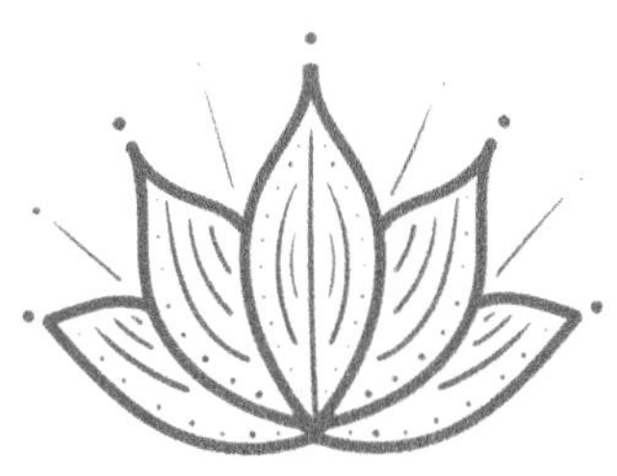

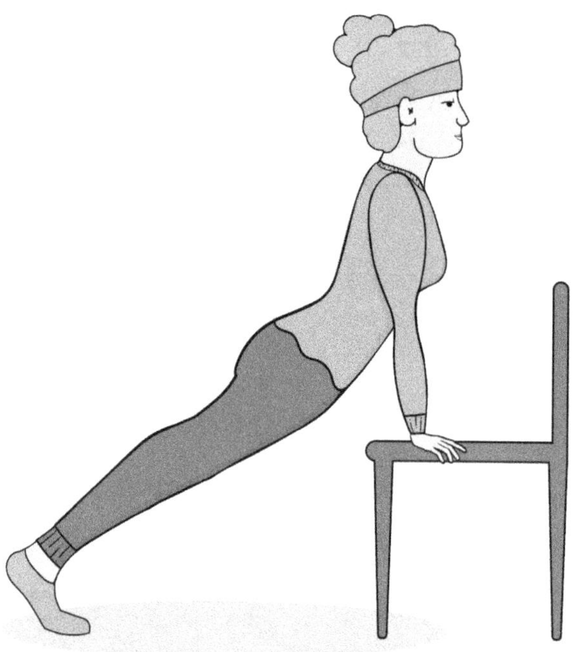

Limitations:

If you have wrist, shoulder, or back pain, you may find it uncomfortable to hold this position, approach with caution and not push yourself too far.

Benefits:

Stretches the chest, shoulders, abdomen, arms, wrist, and legs.

1. Stand facing the chair with your feet just beneath your hip bones' widest point.
2. Firmly put both hands on the chair's seat, keeping your palms facing down.
3. Inhale and lift your chest, drawing your shoulders down and back.
4. Gently press your hands into the chair, keeping your arms straight.
5. Exhale and put your legs behind you.
6. Keep your legs straight and engaged, distributing your weight properly between both feet.
7. Hold the pose for 4 deep breaths.
8. To come out of the pose, inhale and slowly walk your feet towards the chair until you are standing upright again.

32B Variation for People with Wrist Issues

Perform this pose using a chair with armrests to provide extra stability and support or placing a folded blanket on the seat of the chair for additional support and cushioning.

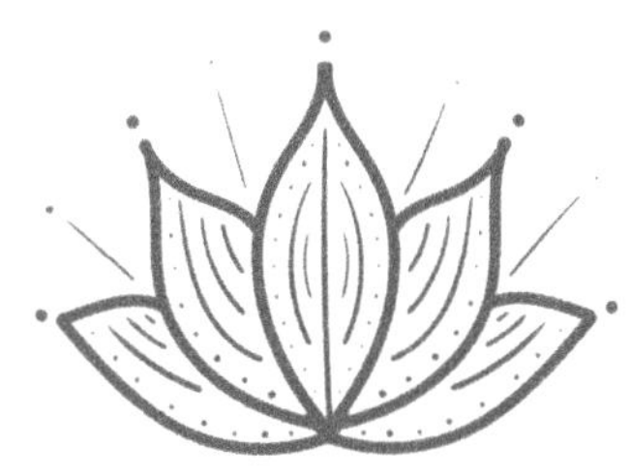

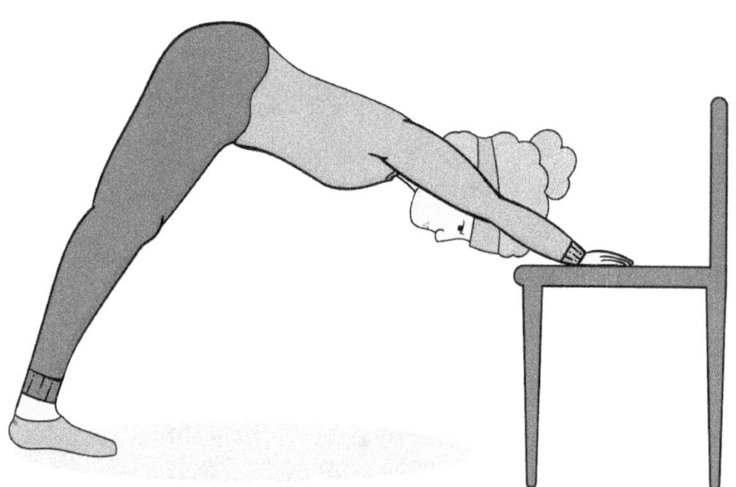

Limitations:

If you have wrist, shoulder, or back pain, you may find this pose uncomfortable. If you have high blood pressure, avoid lowering your head below your heart in this pose.

Benefits:

Stretches the chest, shoulders, abdomen, arms, wrist, and legs.

1. Stand facing the chair with your feet hip-distance apart.

2. Inhale and raise your hands.

3. Exhale and slowly bend forward at the hips, keeping your spine long and your arms straight and bringing your hands to the seat of the chair, keeping your palms facing down.

4. Walk your feet back until your arms and back are parallel to the ground and your hips are over your heels.

5. Keep your head and neck relaxed and your gaze towards your toes or the floor.

6. Press your hands firmly onto the chair's back and engage your arms and upper back muscles. Breathe deeply and hold the pose.

7. To come out of the pose, inhale and slowly walk your feet towards the chair until you are standing upright again.

33B Variation for People with High Blood Pressure

To avoid lowering your head below your heart in this pose. You can use a chair with a higher seat or stack yoga blocks on top of the chair to elevate the hands.

33C Variation to Increase Stretching.

Once you are in the final position, you can bend one knee and extend the other leg back, alternating sides to stretch both hamstrings.

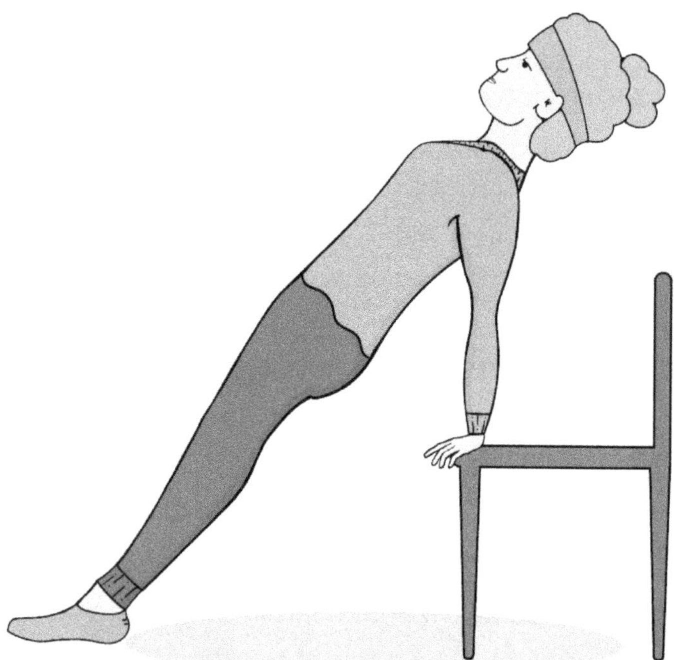

Limitations:

This pose may not be suitable for everyone, especially those with wrist or shoulder injuries or conditions that affect the spine, such as osteoporosis or herniated discs.

Benefits:

Enhances upper body strength, flexibility, and posture and relaxes the chest and shoulders. It can also help with fatigue and minor back discomfort.

1. Begin seated on the chair, facing forward with your hands resting on your thighs.
2. On an inhale, place your hands on the seat of the chair, directly beneath your shoulders.
3. As you exhale, lower your chest down toward the chair, bending your elbows and keeping them close to your body.
4. Inhale, pressing firmly into your hands and straightening your arms, lifting your chest and torso off the chair.
5. Make sure to keep your shoulders relaxed, lowering them.
6. Hold the pose for a few breaths, feeling the stretch in your chest and the engagement in your core.
7. To release, exhale and lower your chest back down to the seat of the chair.
8. Repeat the pose for 3 rounds, moving with your breath.

34B Variation for People with Wrist or Shoulder Issues

For those with wrist or shoulder issues, this pose can be practiced with the forearms resting on the chair seat instead of the hands.

34C Variation to Increase Stretching.

Once you are in the final position, you can bend one knee and extend the other leg back, alternating sides to stretch both hamstrings.

Limitations:

Perform this sequence carefully. Stop it or slow down if you feel pain or discomfort.

Benefits:

Improve flexibility, circulation, and balance, reduce stress, strengthen muscles, and help control weight.

Instructions:

Each movement will be accompanied by inhalation and exhalation.

SEATED PRAYER POSE

1. Sit on your chair, set your feet squarely on the ground and straighten your spine.
2. With your fingers pointing up, bring your palms together near your chest.
3. Press your palms together with gentle pressure.
4. Breathe using your nose.

CHAIR MOUNTAIN (TADASANA)

5. Inhale and raise your arms.

SEATED FORWARD FOLD (UTTANASANA)

6. Exhale and fold forward from your hips, bringing your hands towards your feet. Lengthen the spine and keep your head and shoulders relaxed.

SEATED FORWARD FOLD (ARDHA UTTANASANA)

7. Inhale and come up with your hand on your thighs and your spine straight. Look forward.

8. Exhale and return to the starting pose.

SEATED HAPPY BABY POSE

9. Inhale and lift one of your knees towards your chest and grab it with your hands. Keeping the other foot on the ground.

10. Exhale and bring your lifted leg gently towards your chest.

11. Repeat with the other knee.

12. Come back to the original position.

CHAIR COBRA POSE (BHUJANGASANA)

13. Inhale and lift your chest up, arching your back and keeping your elbows close to your side.

14. Look up and breathe deeply.

FLOWING SEQUENCES

15. Once you finish the first round of this sequence, repeat it 3 to 5 times from steps 5 to 14.

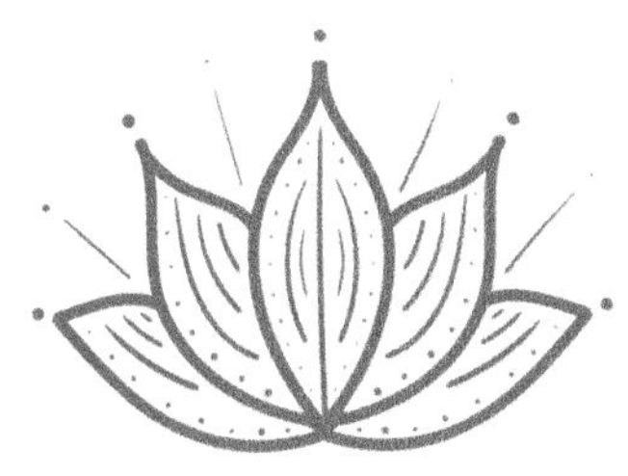

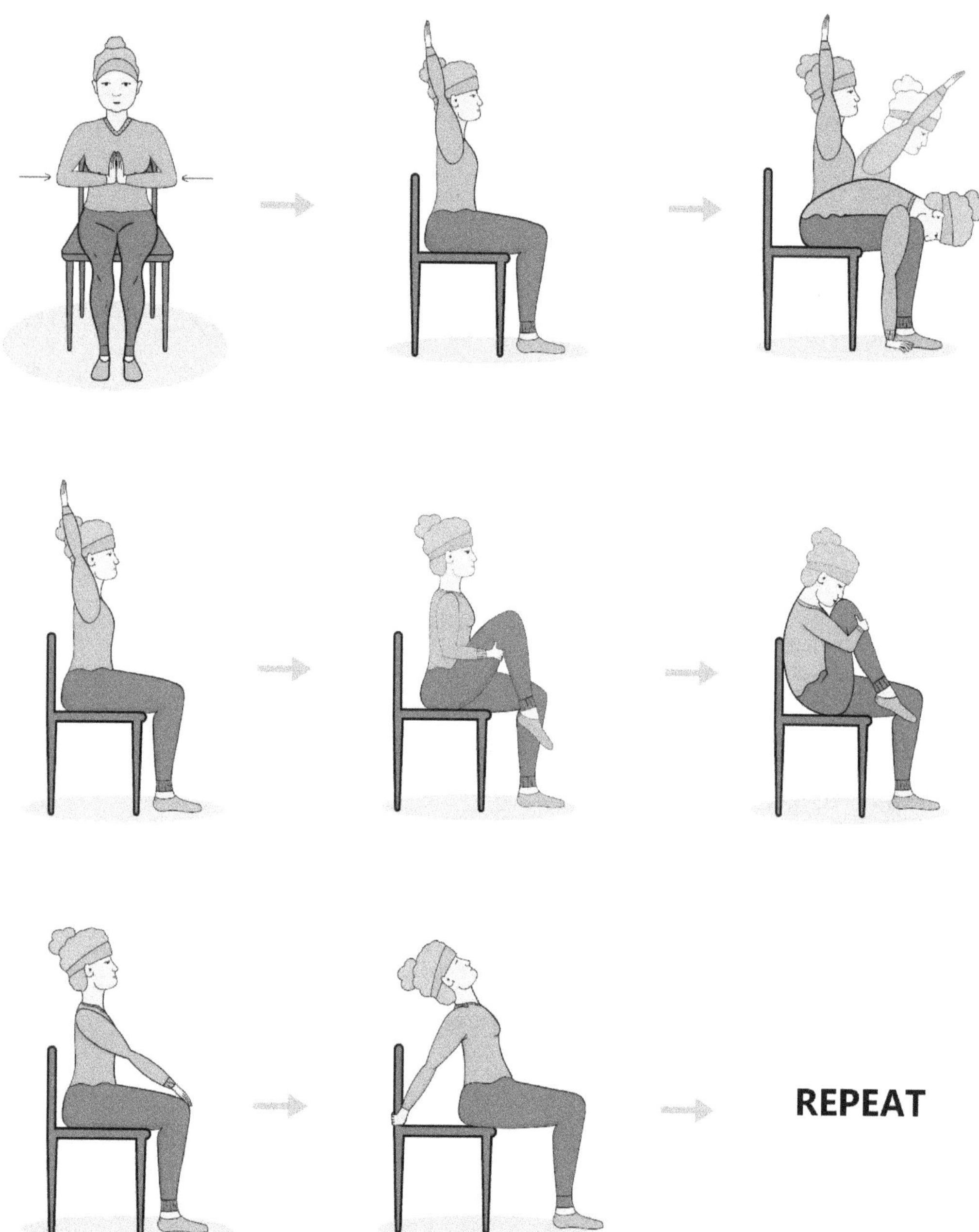

REPEAT

Pranayama: The Power of Breathing

Incorporating Pranayama into one's yoga practice is a fundamental component of enhancing overall health and wellness, widely recognized for its significant and positive impact. Pranayama involves controlling and guiding the act of inhaling and exhaling. Mastery of controlled breathing techniques enables individuals to access many benefits that significantly enhance their physical, mental, and emotional well-being.

Pranayama offers numerous key advantages, notably the ability to enhance the respiratory system's performance. By employing breath regulation techniques and perfecting deep inhalation and exhalation, we can augment the efficacy of oxygen distribution within the organism, subsequently fostering paramount well-being and energy. Moreover, incorporating pranayama practices can augment our potential to achieve attentiveness and concentration, concurrently mitigating the levels of stress and unease.

It is imperative to exercise utmost caution while practicing Pranayama, especially if there are pre-existing medical conditions that may impede physical activity. Always seek guidance from your healthcare professional before initiating a pranayama-based exercise regimen.

Numerous pranayama techniques are available, each offering unique advantages. Some of the most practiced pranayama techniques include:

36 Diaphragmatic Breathing

Deep belly breathing, also known as diaphragmatic breathing, involves taking slow and deep breaths while focusing on expanding the belly instead of the chest. This technique is effective for calming the mind and reducing stress and anxiety. It can also improve oxygen flow in the body, lower blood pressure, and improve digestion. Regular practice might make you feel more energized, focused, and calm.

1. Sit on your chair, straighten your spine, and place your feet firmly on the ground.

2. With your eyes closed, take slow, deep breaths using your nose, and concentrate on your abdomen.

3. Breathe in and let your abdomen expand.

4. Exhale and let your abdomen naturally contract.

5. Try to equalize the length of your inhalation and exhalation, concentrating on the sensation of your breath moving through your body.Sit on your chair, straighten your spine, and place your feet firmly on the ground.

37 Nadi Shodhana Pranayama

This technique involves alternating breathing between the left and right nostrils, believed to balance the brain's hemispheres and clear nasal passages. Nadi Shodhana Pranayama can help balance energy flow in the body, calm the mind and nervous system, enhance respiratory health, and assist with breath control. It is also effective in reducing stress.

Instructions:

1. Sit on your chair, straighten your spine, and place your feet firmly on the ground.

2. Place your right hand near your nose and use your thumb to close your right nostril.

3. Inhale slowly through your left nostril, counting to four.

4. Hold your breath for a count of four.

5. Use your right ring finger to close your left nostril, then open your right nostril.

6. Exhale slowly and fully through your right nostril, counting to eight.

7. Repeat these steps, increasing the count as comfortable.

Also known as equal breathing, this technique involves equalizing the length of inhalation and exhalation, creating a balanced effect on the body and mind. It is helpful in relieving pain, reducing anxiety, and adaptable for different ability levels.

Instructions:

1. Find a comfortable seated position.

2. Take a few deep breaths to center and relax your body.

3. Inhale slowly through your nose for a count of four.

4. Hold your breath for a count of four.

5. Exhale completely through your nose for a count of four.

6. Hold your breath again for a count of four.

7. Repeat this cycle for several minutes, gradually increasing the count as comfortable

39 Kapalabhati Pranayama

This technique involves rapid, forceful exhalations and is thought to clear the lungs and respiratory passages, as well as tone the abdominal muscles. Kapalabhati Pranayama stimulates abdominal organs, improves digestion, increases lung capacity, and can clear nasal passages. However, it should be avoided by people with high blood pressure, heart problems, respiratory disorders, or any condition aggravated by forceful breathing.

Instructions:

1. Sit on your chair, straighten your spine, and cross your legs.

2. Take a few deep breaths to center and relax your body.

3. Begin by inhaling deeply, filling your lungs with air.

4. Exhale vigorously, contracting your abdominal muscles towards your spine

to expel the air.

5. Inhale passively, allowing your belly to expand.

6. Repeat this process in quick succession, creating a rhythm and pumping the breath out through your nose.

7. Start with a few rounds of 10-20 breaths, gradually building up to longer sets.

8. After completing the practice, take time to sit quietly and pay attention to any sensations in your body.

Relaxation (Savasana), Gratitude & Meditation

To properly end your practice, include the following sequence in your routine. This sequence constitutes the last step of our 7-step Chair Yoga Routine

40 Savasana

1. While deeply Breathing, start scanning your body from top to bottom, noticing any areas of tension or discomfort.

2. Become aware of the sensation of your breath entering and leaving your body as you bring your focus back to breathing.

3. With each exhalation, let all the tension and stress leave your body.

4. Repeat as long as you like.

5. Conclude your practice, expressing gratitude aloud.

I am grateful for /to ...

6. If you have time and want to include an important component of Yoga Lifestyle in your daily Practice, Meditate for at least 5 minutes.

This 10-minute chair yoga sequence is uniquely tailored for seniors, especially those focused on weight loss and enhancing overall well-being, including beginners, or those with limited mobility or balance concerns. The routine is thoughtfully designed to be accessible, focusing primarily on seated yoga exercises that are easy to follow yet effective for a quick workout. The sequence comprises:

Gentle but Effective Movements: These exercises aim to stimulate metabolism, aiding in weight management and muscle toning.

Calorie-Burning Focus: Despite being seated, the exercises are structured to burn calories, crucial for weight loss.

Flexibility and Stability Enhancement: Through targeted movements, the sequence improves flexibility and stability, essential for senior health.

Cognitive Stimulation: The focus required for yoga poses can also enhance mental clarity and concentration.

Quick and Convenient: Only 10 minutes long, it's perfect for busy schedules or those who prefer shorter exercise sessions.

This inclusive, senior-friendly chair yoga sequence offers a harmonious blend of physical and mental health benefits, making it an excellent choice for seniors looking to stay active and healthy.

Total Duration: 10 minutes

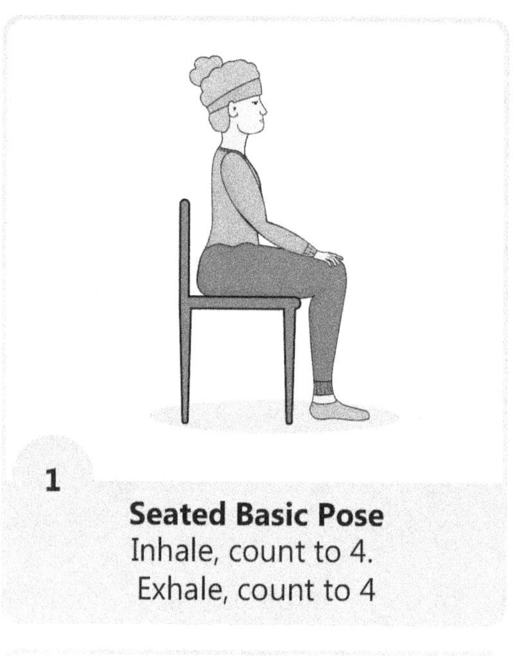

1

Seated Basic Pose
Inhale, count to 4.
Exhale, count to 4

Express your intention
aloud starting with:

I intend to ...
I am ... (or)
I want to ...

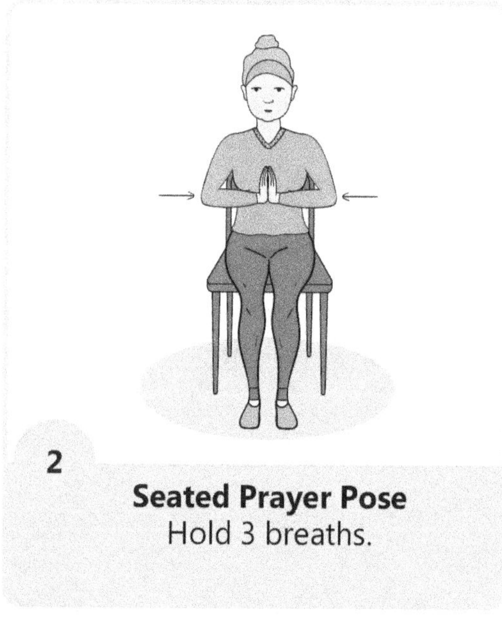

2

Seated Prayer Pose
Hold 3 breaths.

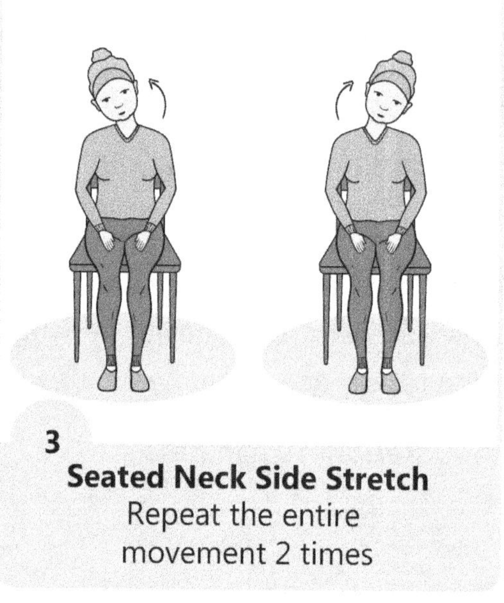

3

Seated Neck Side Stretch
Repeat the entire
movement 2 times

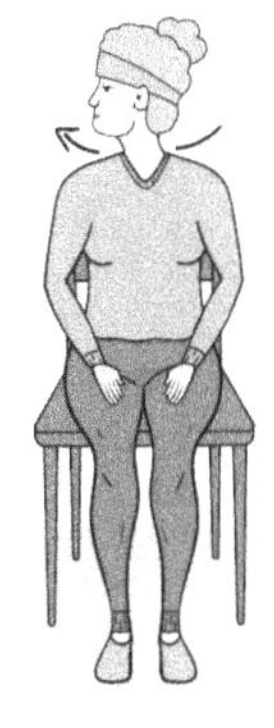

4

Seated Neck Roll
Repeat 2-time for
each direction

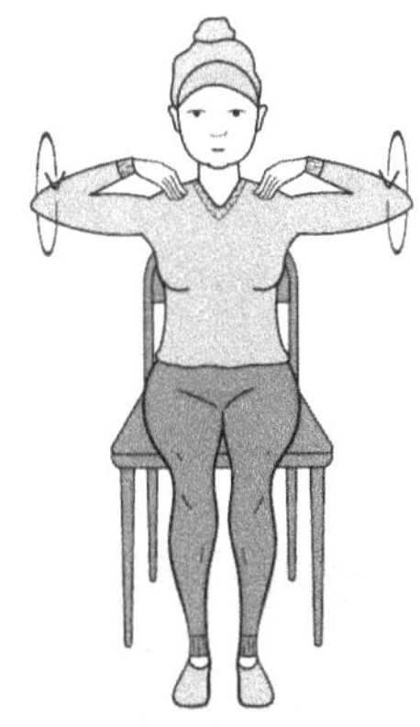

5

Seated Shoulder Roll
Repeat 2-time for
each direction

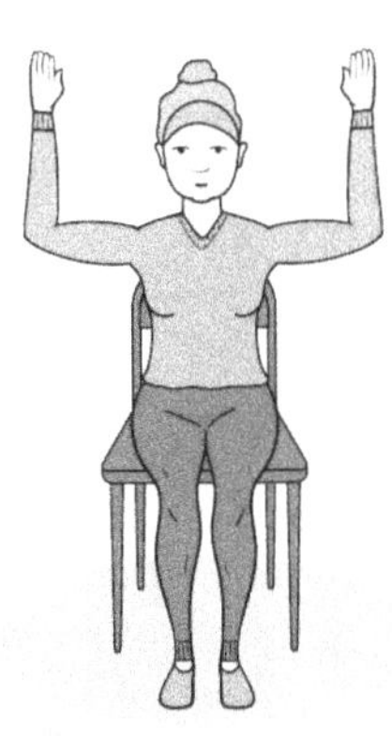
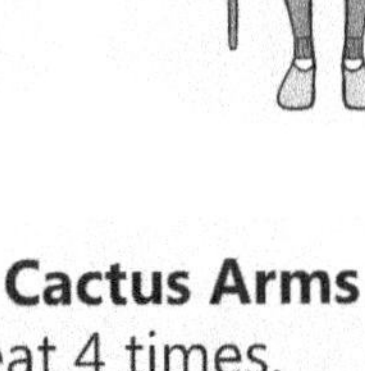

6

Seated Cactus Arms
Repeat 4 times.

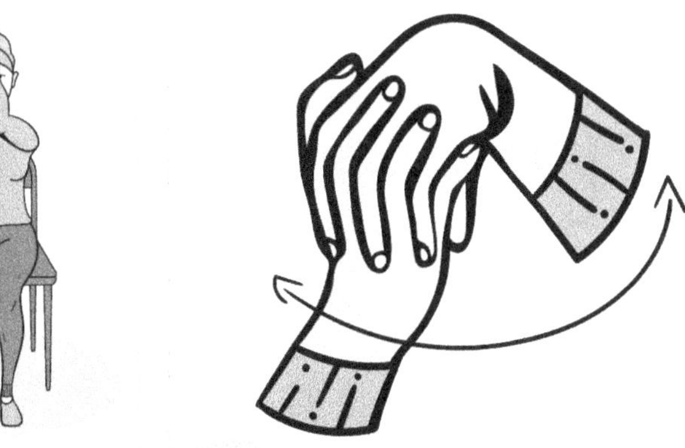

10

Wrist Circle Yoga
Repeat 3-times clockwise
and switch direction

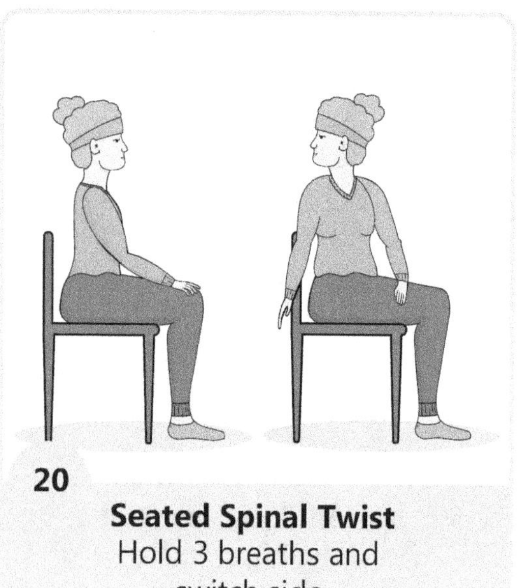

20
Seated Spinal Twist
Hold 3 breaths and
switch side.

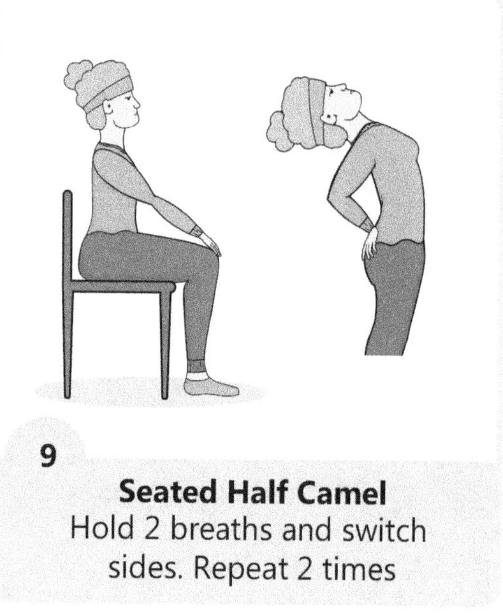

9
Seated Half Camel
Hold 2 breaths and switch
sides. Repeat 2 times

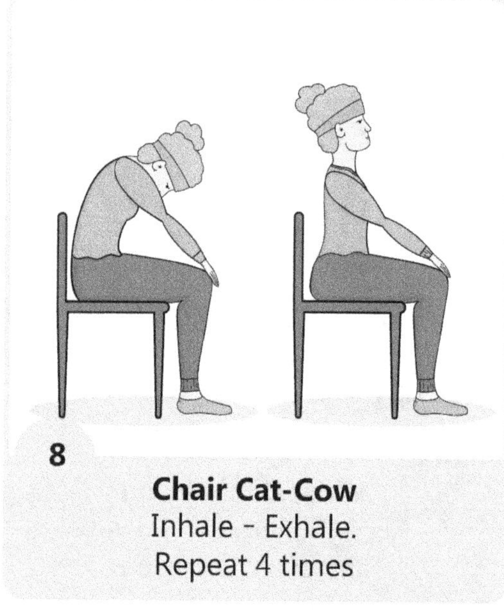

8
Chair Cat-Cow
Inhale – Exhale.
Repeat 4 times

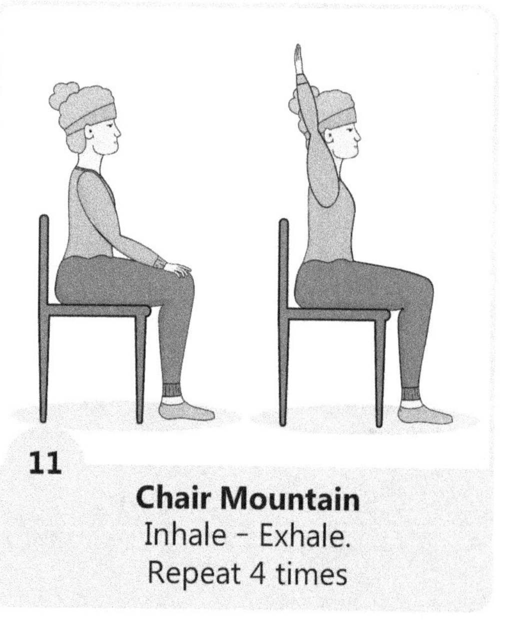

11
Chair Mountain
Inhale – Exhale.
Repeat 4 times

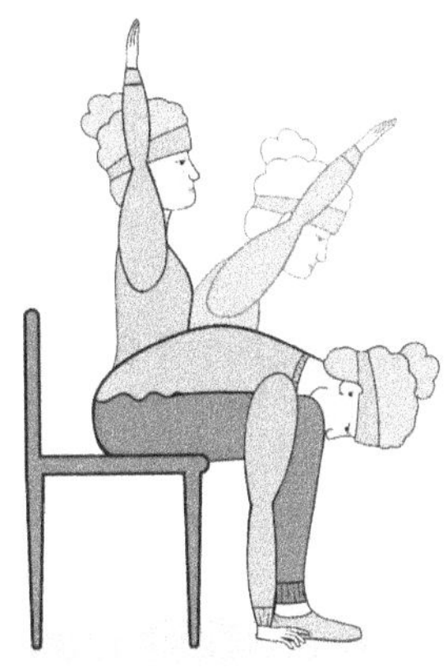

Seated Forward Fold
Inhale – Exhale.
Repeat 2 times

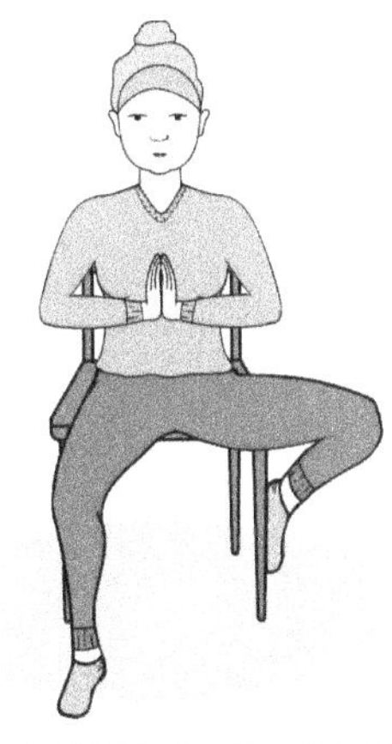

Chair Tree
Hold 2 breaths
and switch sides.

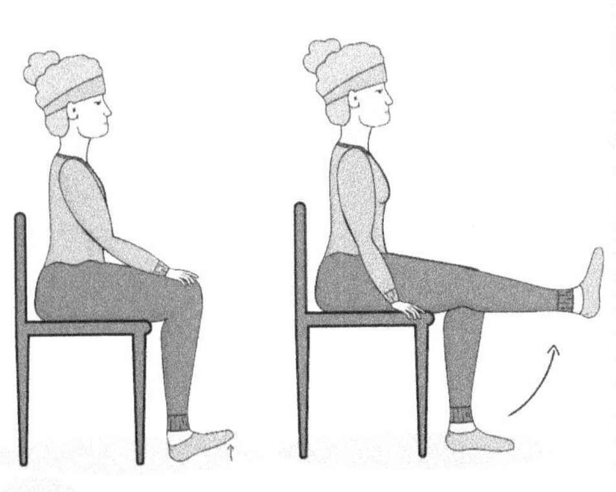

Seated Toe Lifts & Taps
Hold 4 breaths
and switch side.

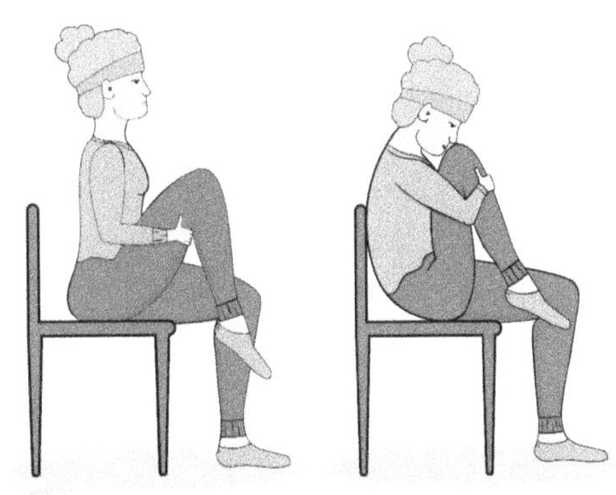

Seated Happy Baby Pose
Hold 3 breaths
and switch leg.

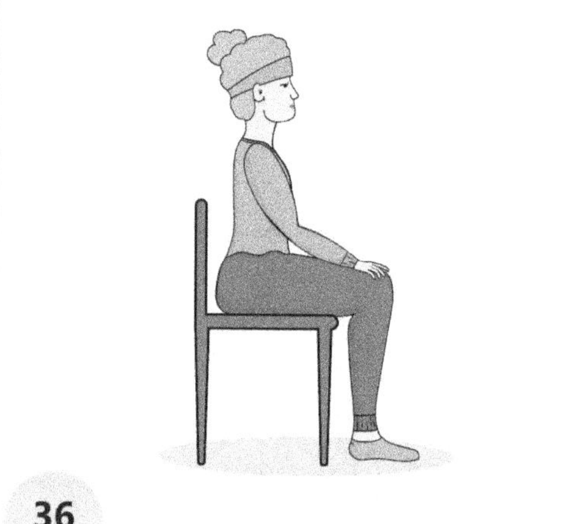

36

Diaphragmatic Breathing
Inhale and exhale equalizing
breathing time.

Conclude your practice,
expressing gratitude aloud:

I am grateful for /to ...

Meditate 5 minutes (optional)

40

Savasana
Breathe, be grateful and
meditate.

This 15-minute intermediate chair yoga sequence, ideal for seniors, goes beyond mere weight loss and fitness enhancement. It incorporates a blend of dynamic, standing, and seated poses, targeting muscle strength, flexibility, and balance, crucial for daily function and fall prevention. Key benefits of this routine include:

Muscle Strengthening and Toning: Focusing on major muscle groups, the sequence aids in building strength, essential for everyday activities.

Improved Flexibility: Regular practice increases joint and muscle flexibility, reducing the risk of injuries and aiding mobility.

Metabolic Enhancement: The dynamic poses help boost metabolism, facilitating more effective weight management.

Balance and Coordination: Essential for fall prevention in seniors, these exercises improve bodily coordination.

Enhanced Circulation: The routine promotes better blood flow, ensuring efficient oxygen and nutrient distribution.

Stress Reduction: Incorporates stress-relieving breathing and relaxation techniques, promoting mental clarity and calmness.

Before starting, seniors should consult healthcare providers to align the routine with their health status and goals.

Total Duration: 15 minutes

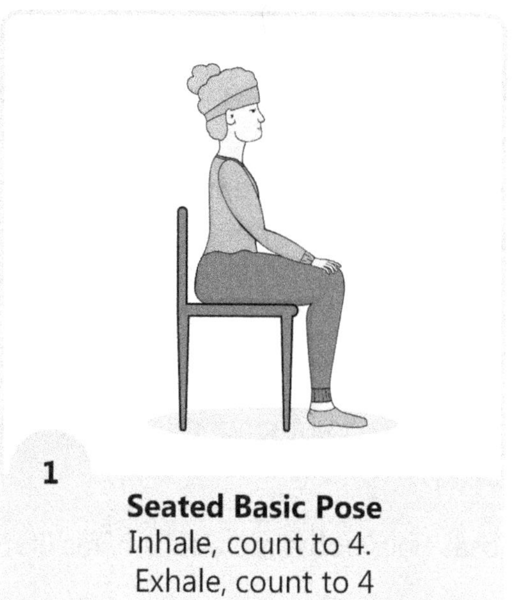

1

Seated Basic Pose
Inhale, count to 4.
Exhale, count to 4

Express your intention
aloud starting with:

I intend to …
I am … (or)
I want to …

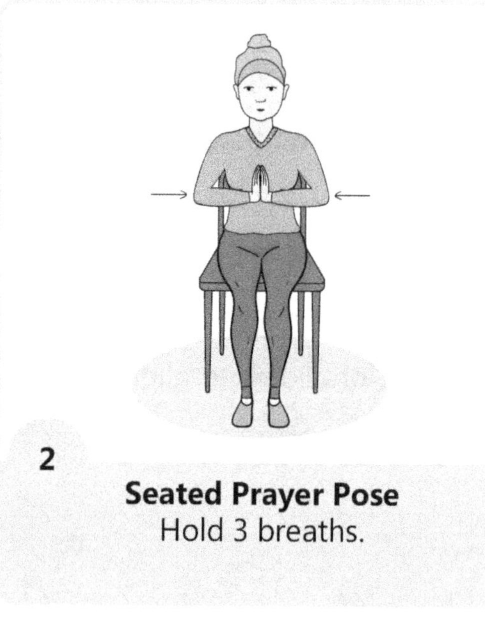

2

Seated Prayer Pose
Hold 3 breaths.

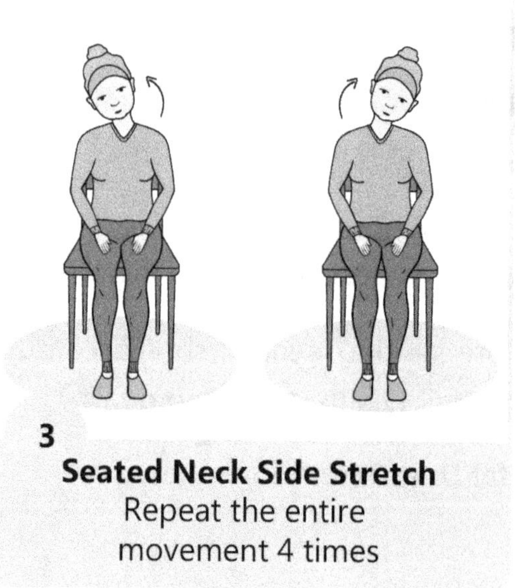

3

Seated Neck Side Stretch
Repeat the entire
movement 4 times

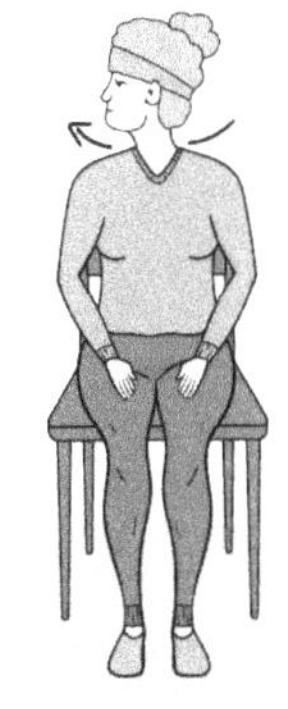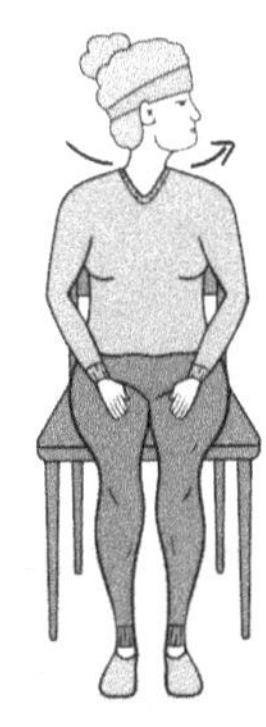

4

Seated Neck Roll
Repeat 2-time for
each direction

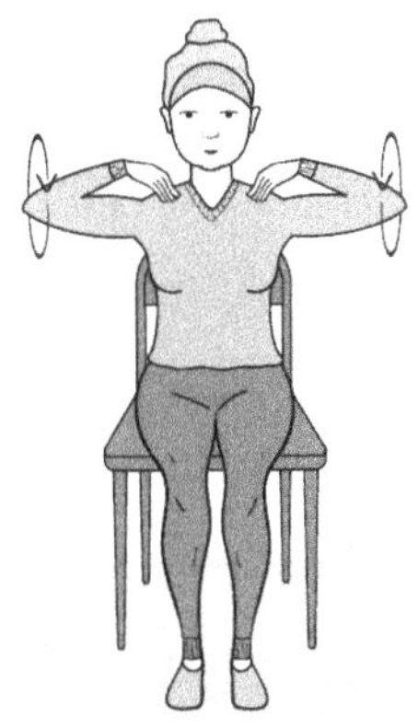

5

Seated Shoulder Roll
Repeat 4-time for
each direction

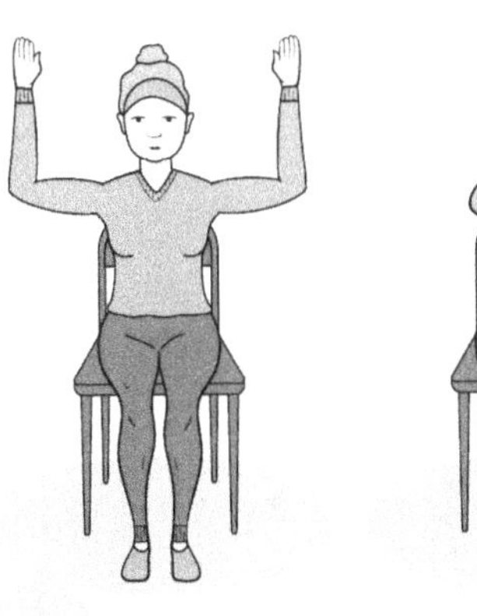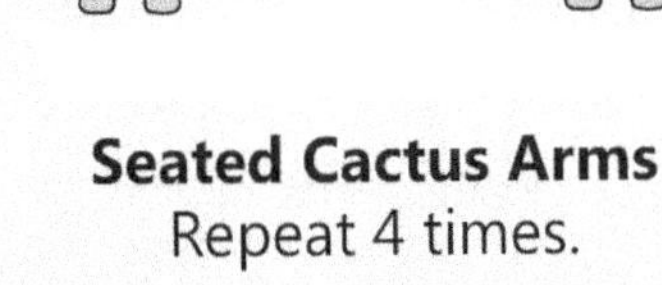

6

Seated Cactus Arms
Repeat 4 times.

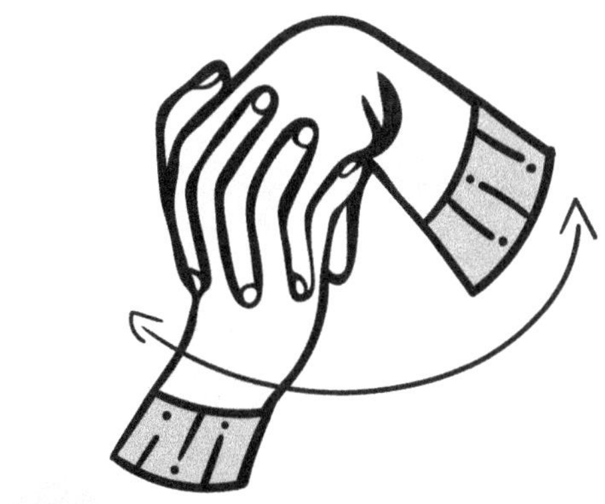

10

Wrist Circle Yoga
Repeat 4-times clockwise
and switch direction

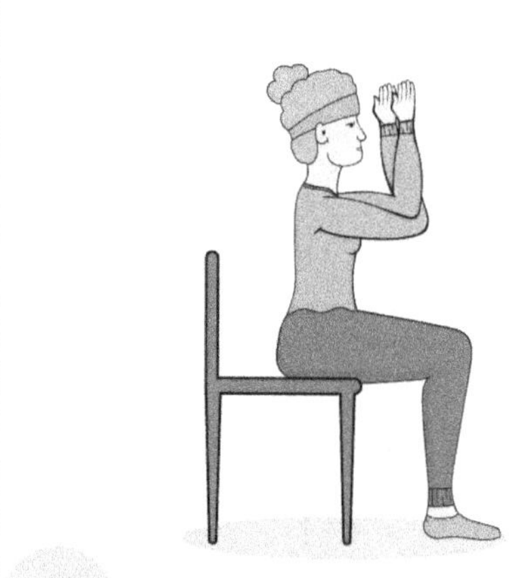

28

Seated Eagle Arms

Hold 4 breaths and switch sides.
Repeat 3 times.

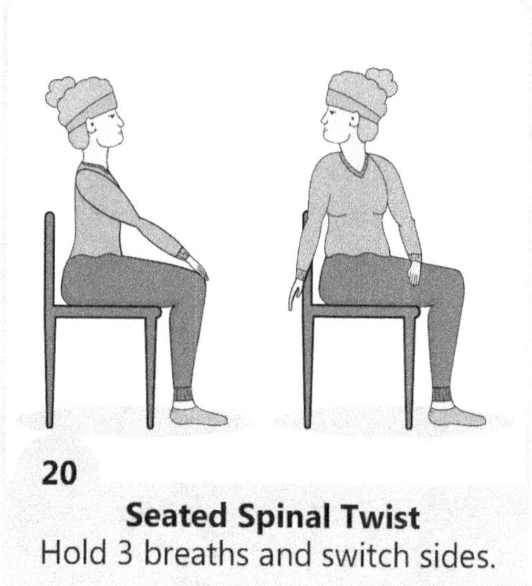

20

Seated Spinal Twist

Hold 3 breaths and switch sides.

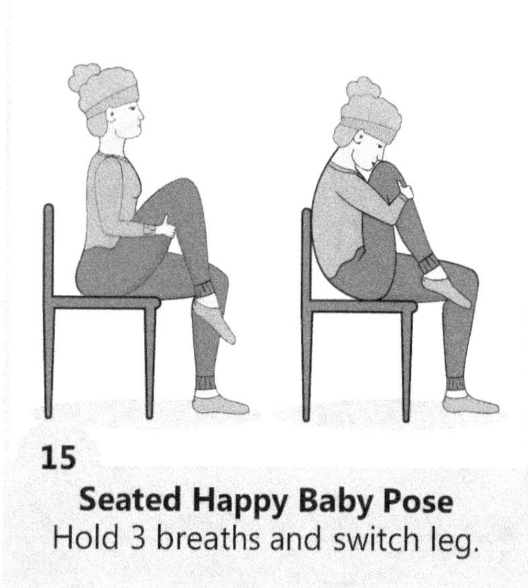

15

Seated Happy Baby Pose

Hold 3 breaths and switch leg.

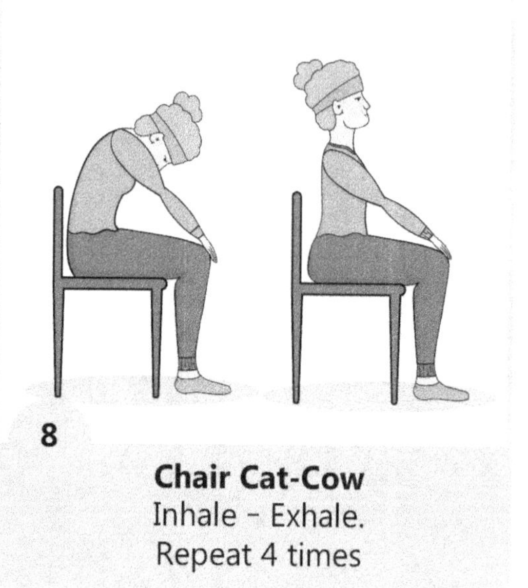

8

Chair Cat-Cow

Inhale – Exhale.
Repeat 4 times

34   **Flowing Sequence**

Each inhalation and exhalation will be accompanied by a movement.

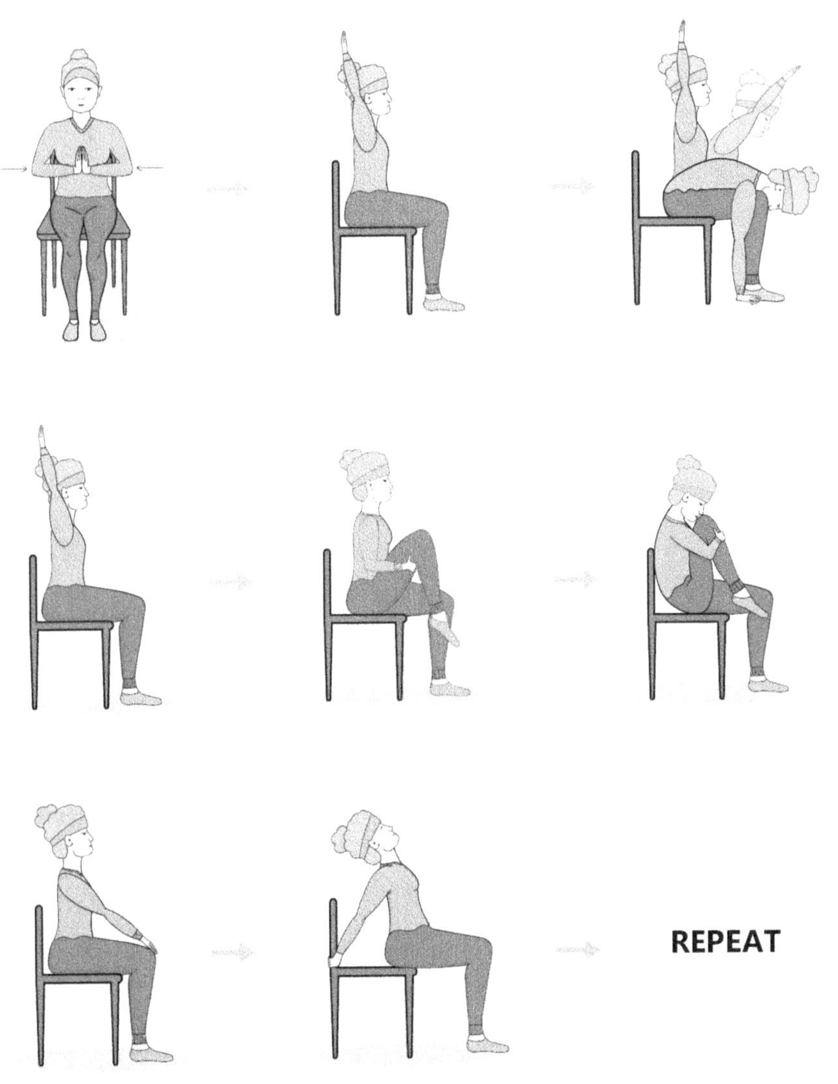

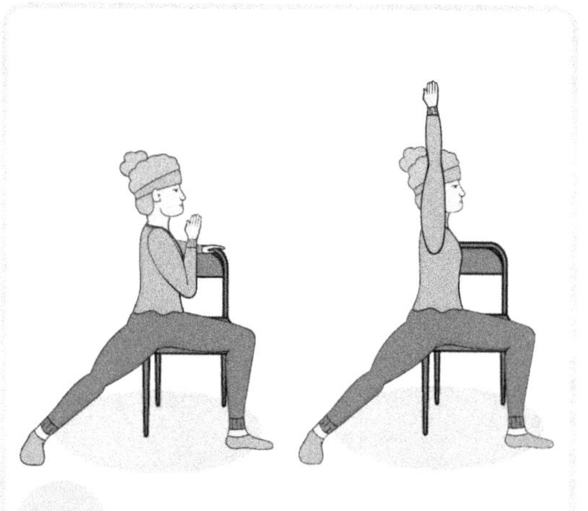

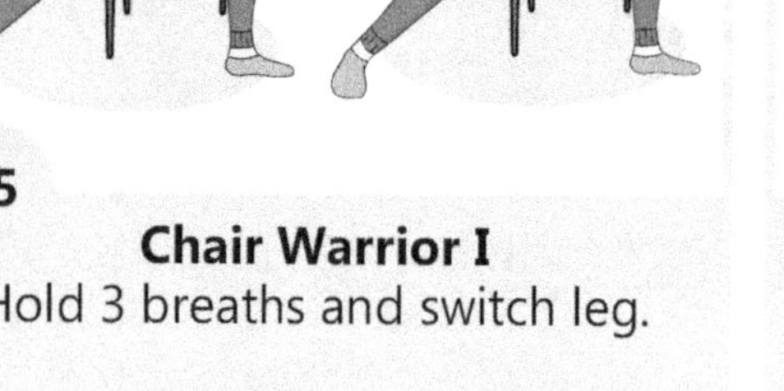

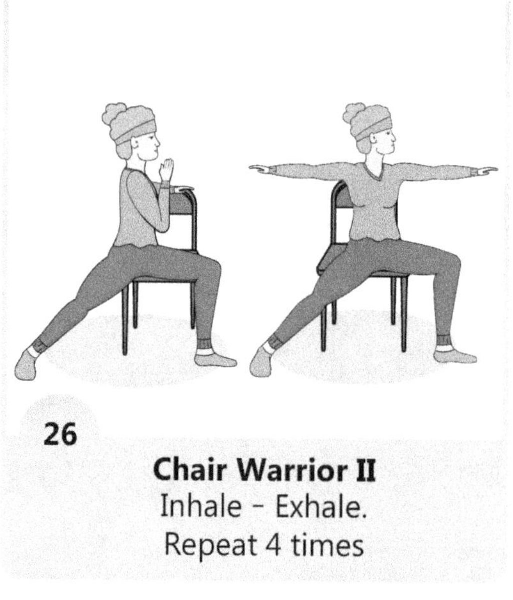

25

Chair Warrior I
Hold 3 breaths and switch leg.

26

Chair Warrior II
Inhale - Exhale.
Repeat 4 times

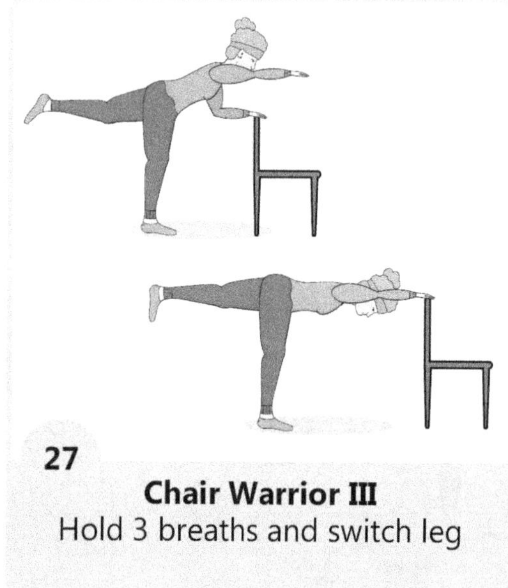

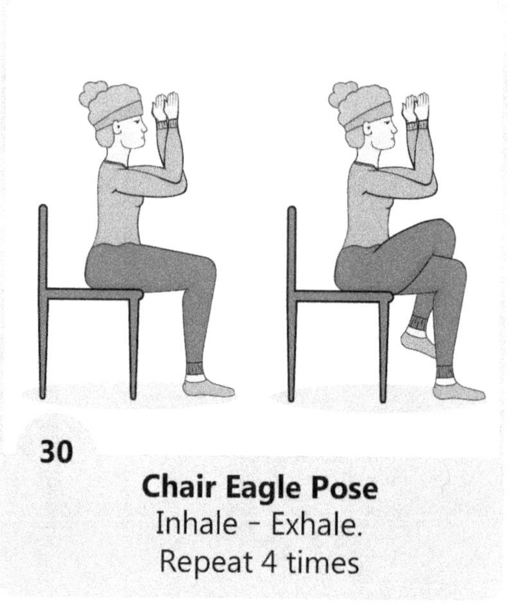

27

Chair Warrior III
Hold 3 breaths and switch leg

30

Chair Eagle Pose
Inhale - Exhale.
Repeat 4 times

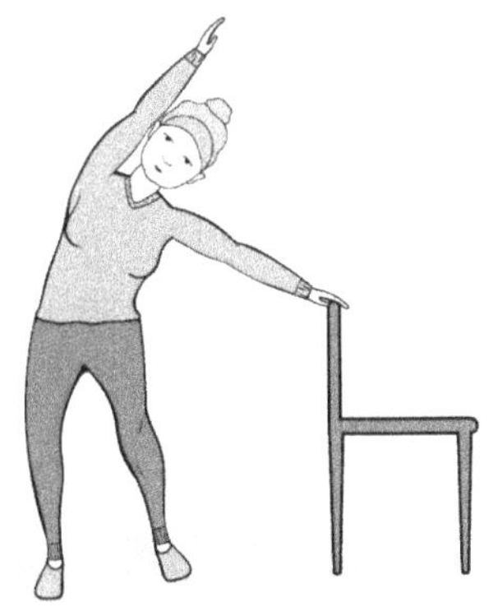

21
Seated Eagle Arms
Hold 3 breaths and switch leg.

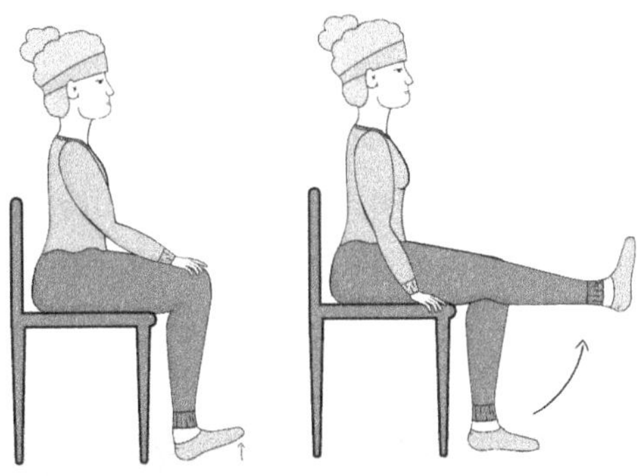

14
Seated Toe Lifts & Taps
Hold 4 breaths and switch side.

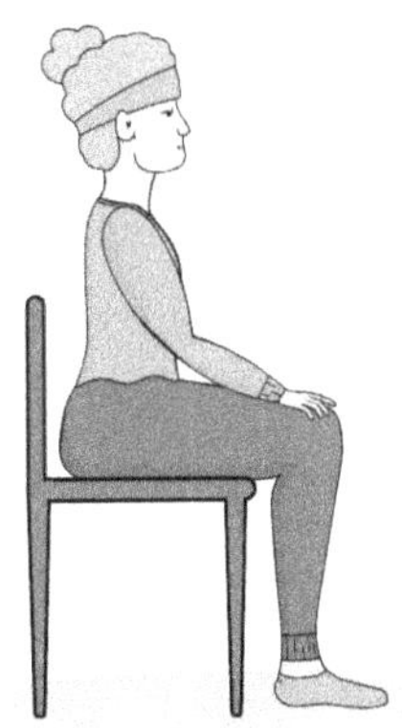

37
Nadi Shodhana
Inhale using one nostril, hold
and exhale using the other

Conclude your practice,
expressing gratitude aloud:

I am grateful for /to ...

Meditate 8 minutes.

40
Savasana
Breathe, be grateful and
meditate.

This 20-minute chair yoga routine is specifically crafted for seniors who aim to integrate yoga into their weight loss plan. The sequence features pose that focus on strengthening and stretching the body, enhancing metabolism, boosting blood circulation, and fostering relaxation and mental clarity. Each pose is selected to provide a balanced workout that not only aids in weight management but also promotes overall physical and mental well-being.

In this routine, seniors will engage in a series of exercises starting with gentle warm-ups to prepare the body, followed by a mix of seated and standing yoga poses. These poses are designed to activate various muscle groups, helping to build strength and flexibility. Additionally, the routine includes breathing exercises (pranayama) to enhance lung capacity and aid in relaxation, improving focus and mental clarity.

The session concludes with a short meditation or relaxation technique, allowing seniors to assimilate the benefits of the practice, promoting a sense of calm and balance.

It's essential for participants, especially those with pre-existing health conditions, to consult a healthcare professional before beginning this or any new exercise program, to ensure it aligns with their health needs and fitness goals.

Duration: 20 minutes

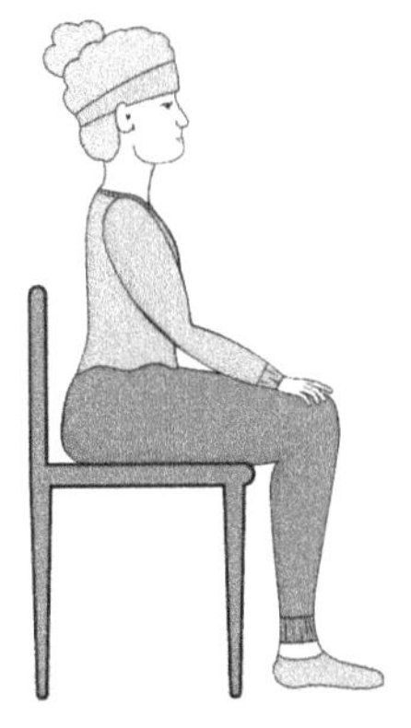

Express your intention aloud starting with:

I intend to ...
I am ... (or)
I want to ...

1

Seated Basic Pose
Inhale, count to 4.
Exhale, count to 4

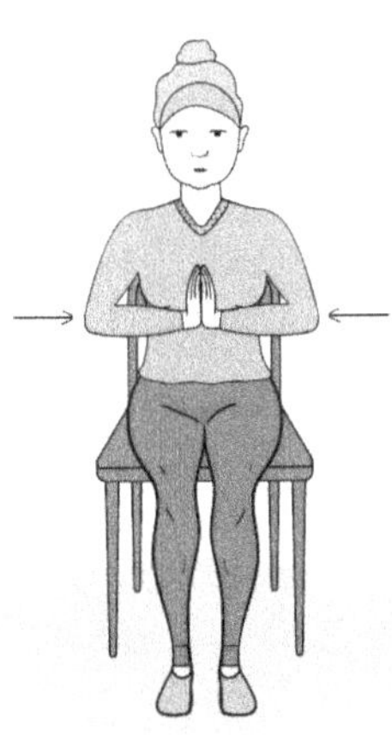

2

Seated Prayer Pose
Hold 4 breaths.

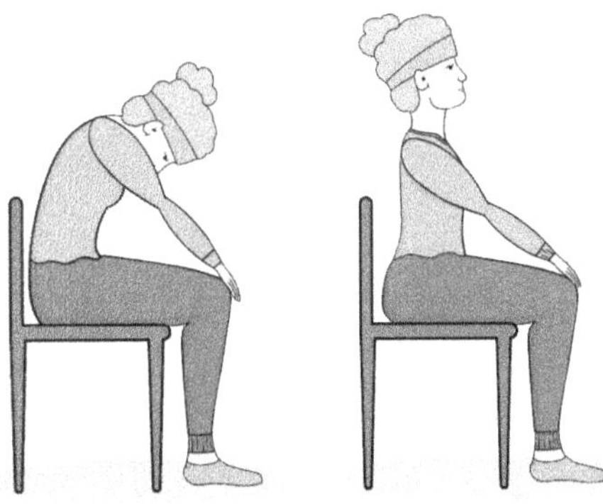

8

Chair Cat-Cow
Inhale - Exhale.
Repeat 4 times

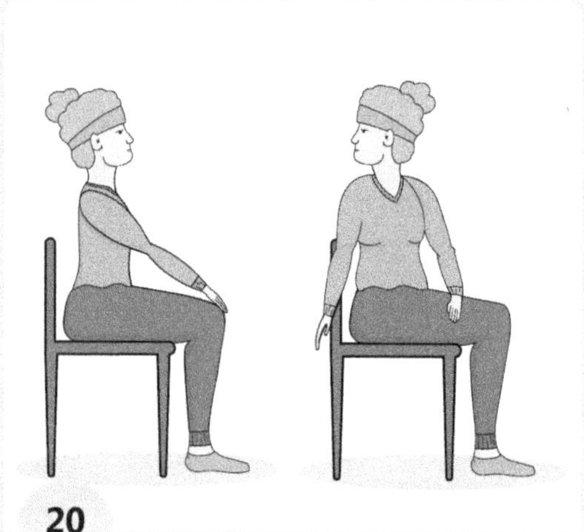

20

Seated Spinal Twist
Hold 3 breaths and switch sides.

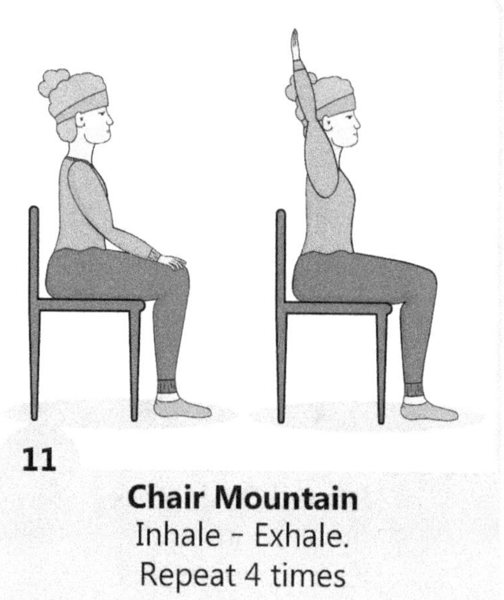

11

Chair Mountain
Inhale – Exhale.
Repeat 4 times

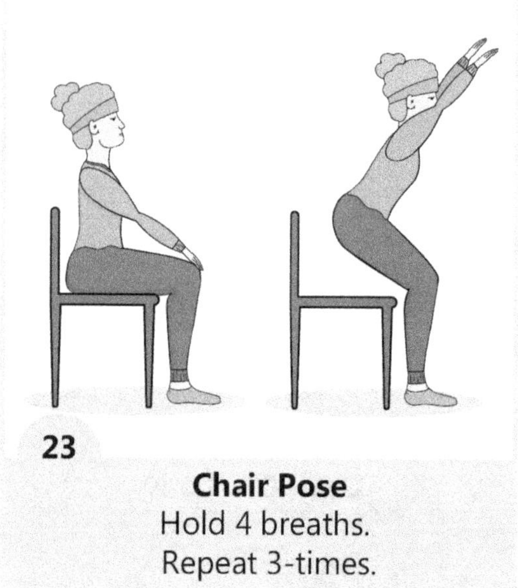

23

Chair Pose
Hold 4 breaths.
Repeat 3-times.

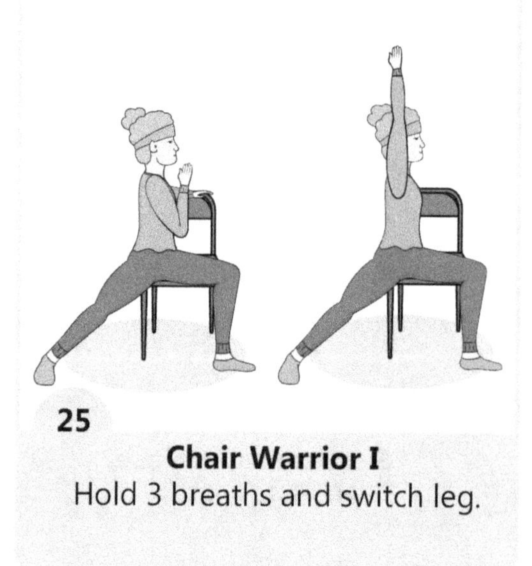

25

Chair Warrior I
Hold 3 breaths and switch leg.

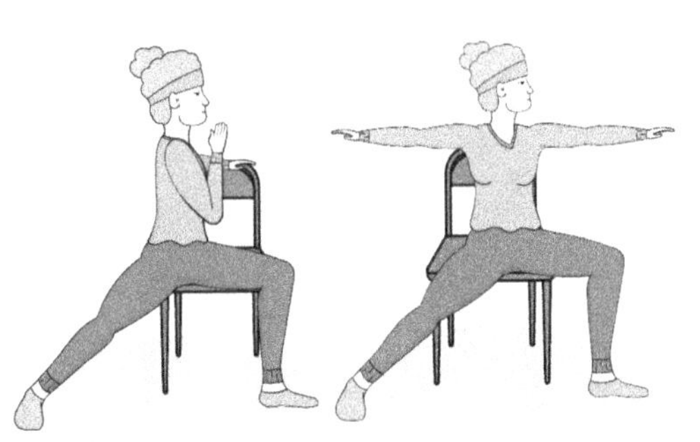

26

Chair Warrior II
Inhale – Exhale.
Repeat 4 times

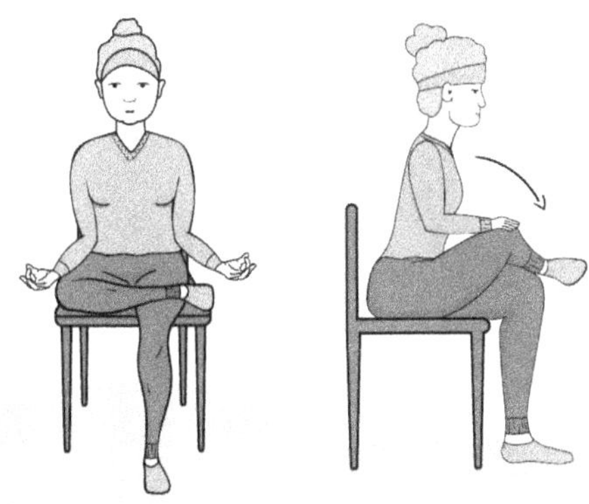

22

Chair Pigeon Pose
Hold 3 breaths and switch sides.

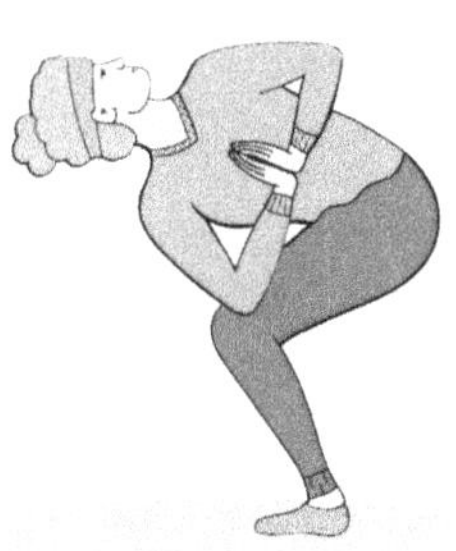

31

Chair Crescent Lunge
Hold 4 breaths and switch sides.
Repeat 3-times.

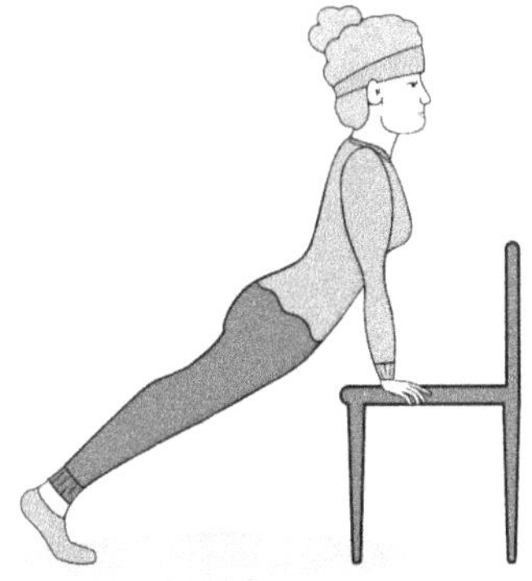

32

Chair Upward-Facing Dog
Hold 3 breaths. Repeat 3-times.

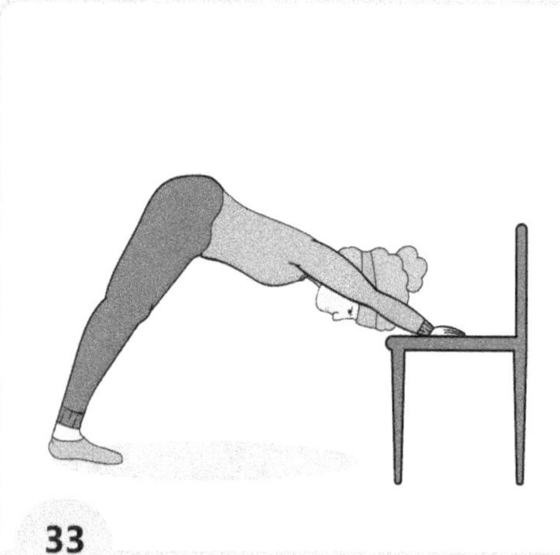

33
Downward-Facing Dog
Hold 4 breaths Repeat 3-times.

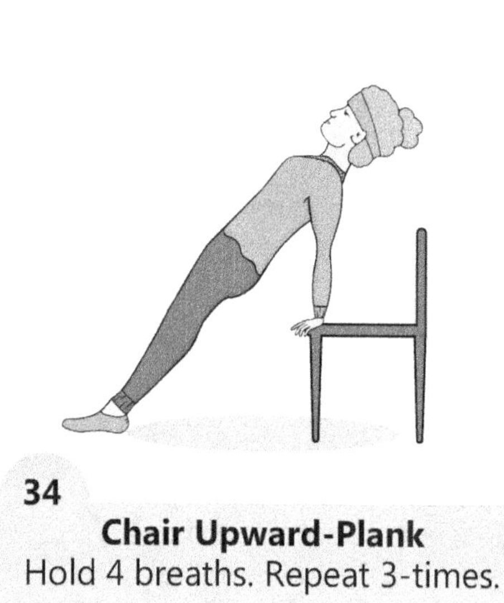

34
Chair Upward-Plank
Hold 4 breaths. Repeat 3-times.

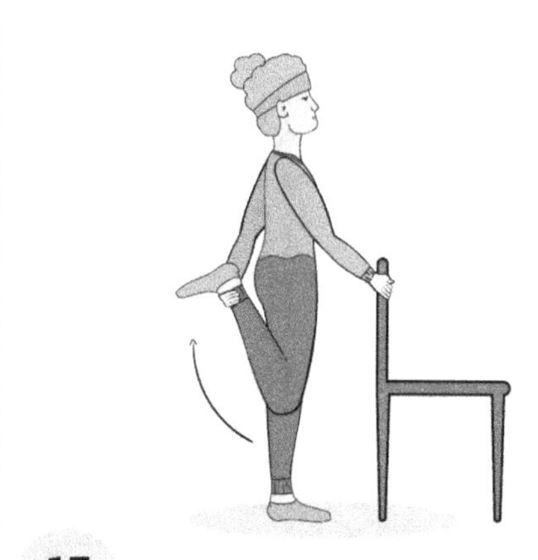

17
Standing Squat Stretch
Hold 3 breaths and switch sides.
Repeat 3-times.

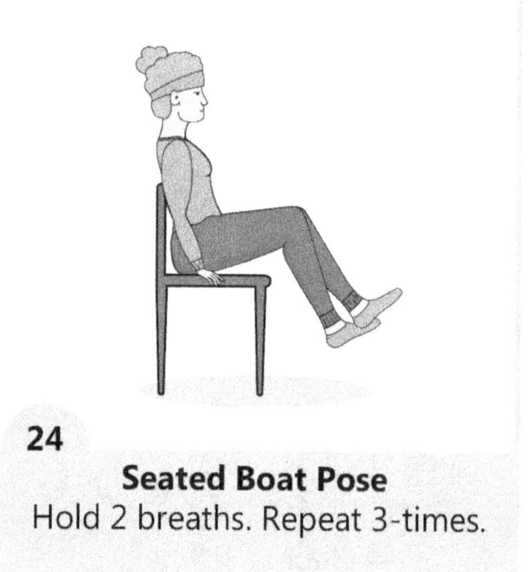

24
Seated Boat Pose
Hold 2 breaths. Repeat 3-times.

 ## Flowing Sequence

Each inhalation and exhalation will be accompanied by a movement.

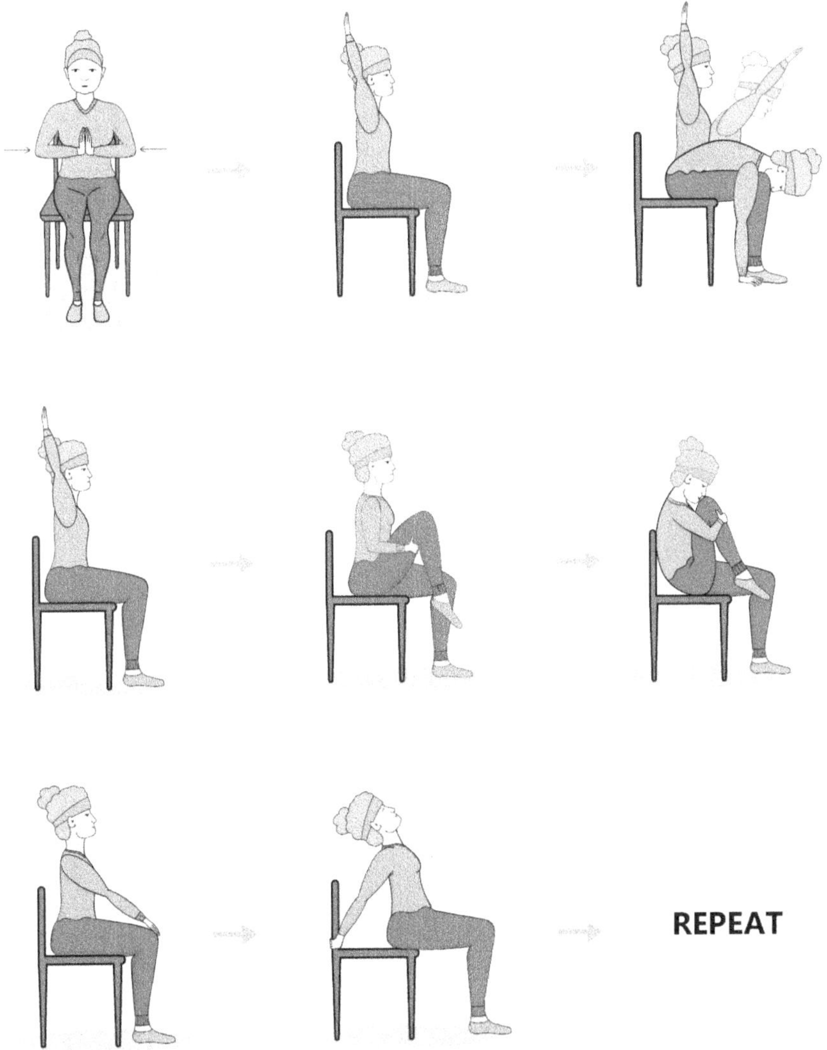

REPEAT

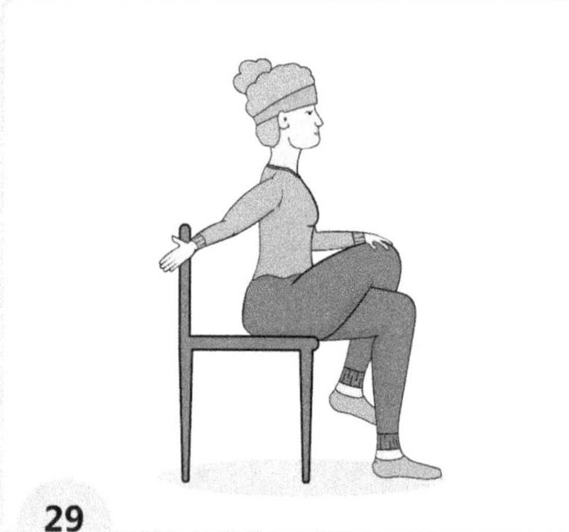

29

Chair Eagle Legs
Hold 2 breaths and switch leg.
Repeat 3-times.

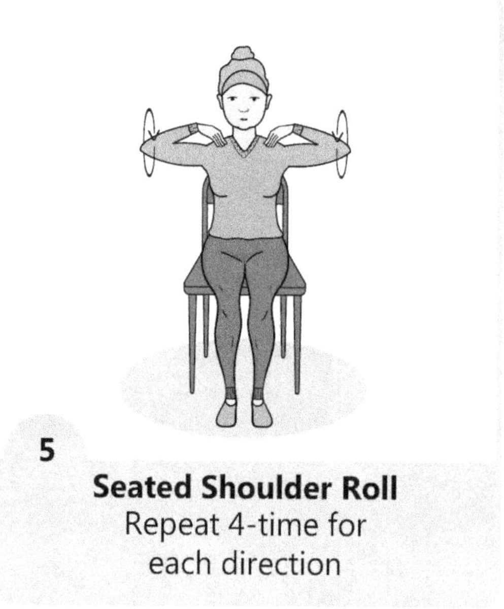

5

Seated Shoulder Roll
Repeat 4-time for
each direction

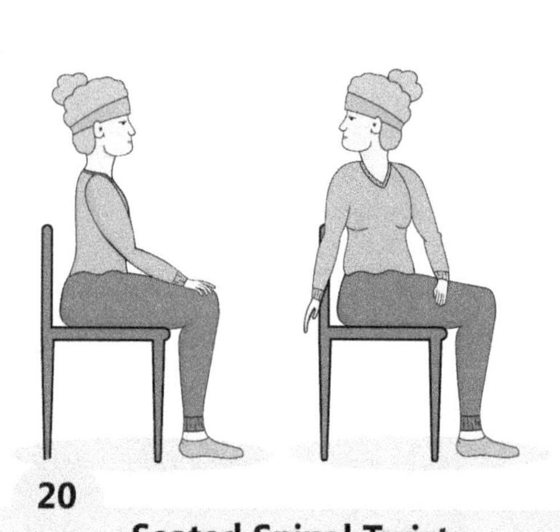

20

Seated Spinal Twist
Hold 3 breaths and switch side.

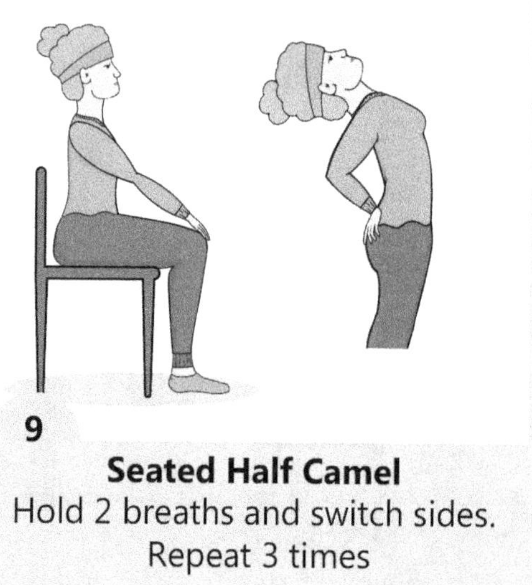

9

Seated Half Camel
Hold 2 breaths and switch sides.
Repeat 3 times

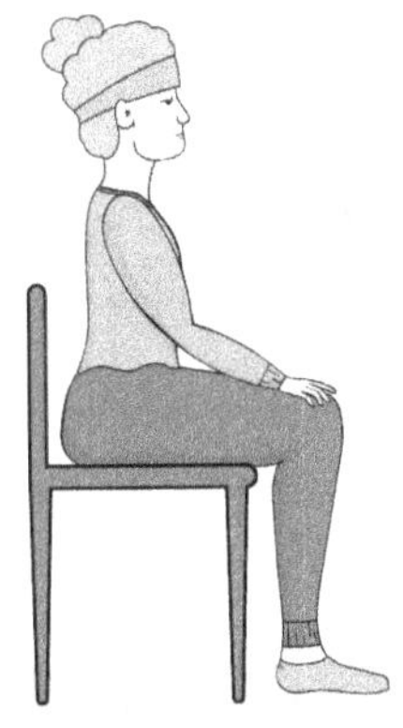

Conclude your practice,
expressing gratitude aloud:

I am grateful for /to ...

Meditate 5 minutes.

39

Kapalabhati Pranayama
Inhale -exhale vigorously.
Repeat 10-times

40

Savasana
Breathe, be grateful and
meditate.

CHAPTER 7: GENTLE ROUTINE FOR SENIORS WITH BONE HEALTH CONCERNS

This 15-minute chair yoga routine is specifically designed for seniors with arthritis, osteoporosis, or low bone density. It emphasizes gentle stretches and movements that are crucial for increasing mobility, flexibility, and muscle strength, while taking care to minimize any risk of injury. Key elements of the routine include:

Gentle Stretching: To ease stiffness in joints and muscles, particularly beneficial for those with arthritis.

Low-Impact Movements: These exercises are safe for individuals with osteoporosis, focusing on strengthening bones without putting undue pressure on them.

Pain Management: The exercises are designed to alleviate discomfort associated with arthritis and similar conditions.

Balance and Stability: Incorporates poses that enhance balance, an essential aspect of preventing falls.

This routine is an excellent way for seniors with specific health concerns to maintain an active lifestyle, improve their physical health, and enhance their overall quality of life. However, it's always advisable to listen to your body and consult a healthcare professional if any discomfort arises.

Total Duration: 15 minutes

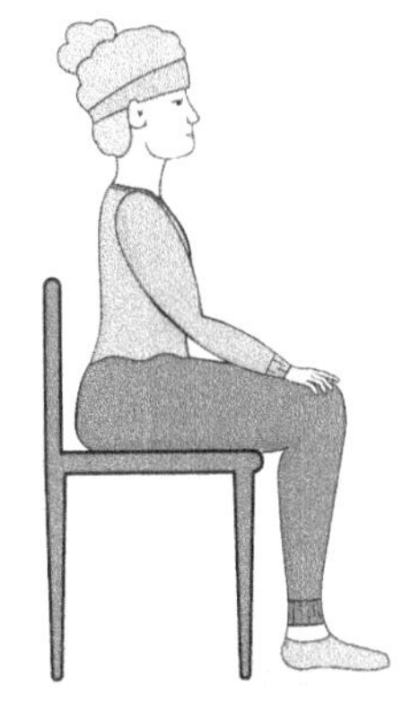

1

Seated Basic Pose
Inhale, count to 4.
Exhale, count to 4

Express your intention aloud starting with:

**I intend to …
I am … (or)
I want to …**

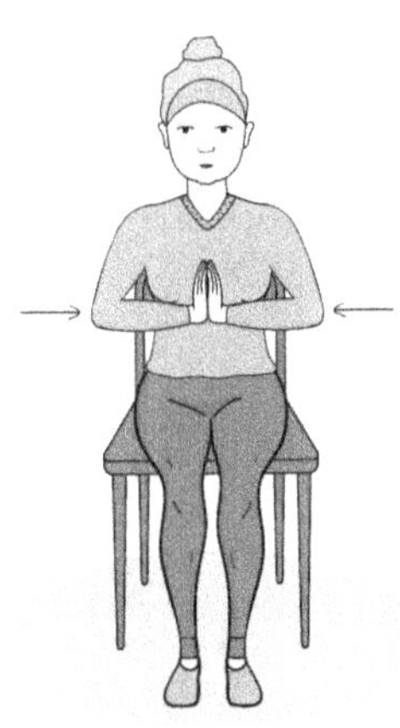

2

Seated Prayer Pose
Hold 4 breaths.

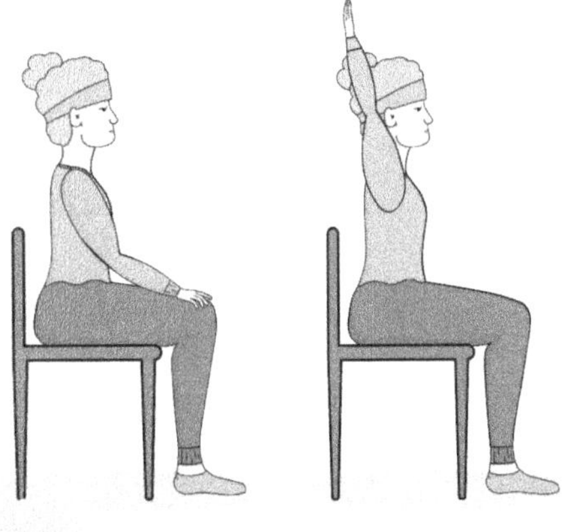

11

Chair Mountain
Inhale – Exhale.
Repeat 4 times

115

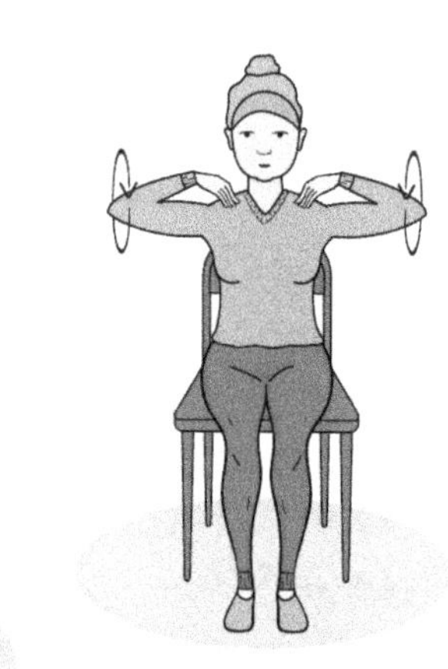

5

Seated Shoulder Roll
Repeat 4-time for
each direction

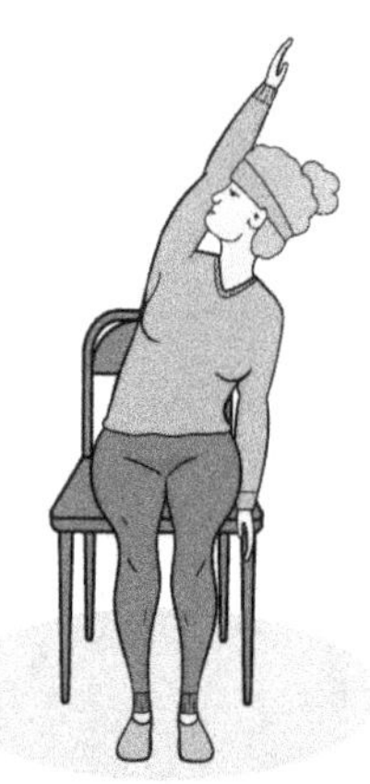

18

Seated Shoulder Roll
Hold 3 breaths and switch sides.
Repeat twice.

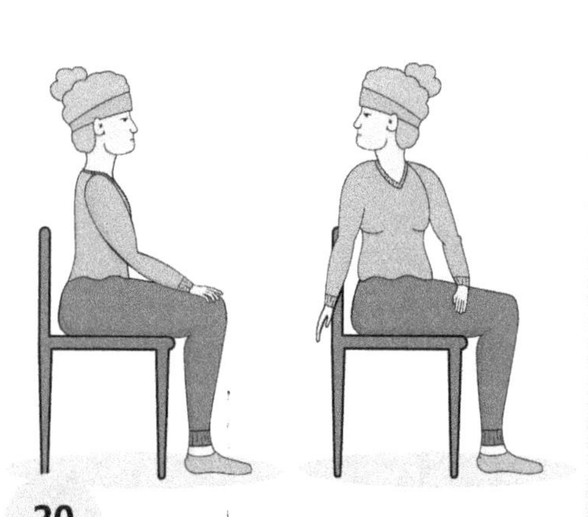

20

Seated Spinal Twist
Hold 3 breaths and switch sides.

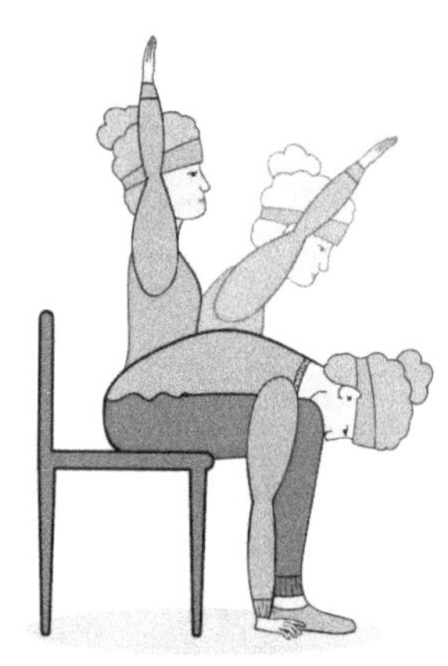

12

Seated Forward Fold
Hold 3 breaths and switch sides.
Repeat 4-times

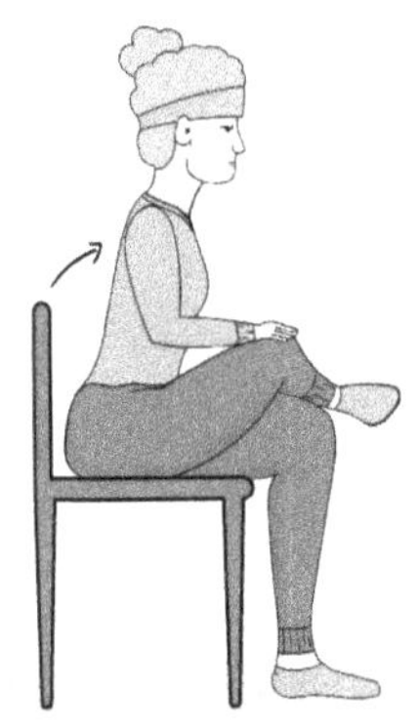

7

Seated Figure Four
Hold 4 breaths and switch sides.

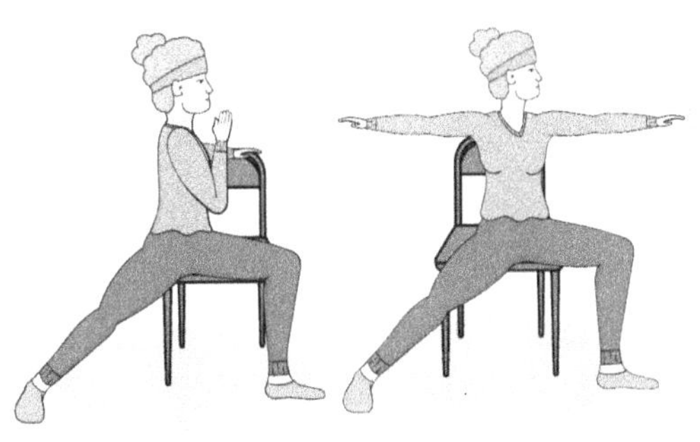

26

Chair Warrior II
Inhale – Exhale.
Repeat 4 times

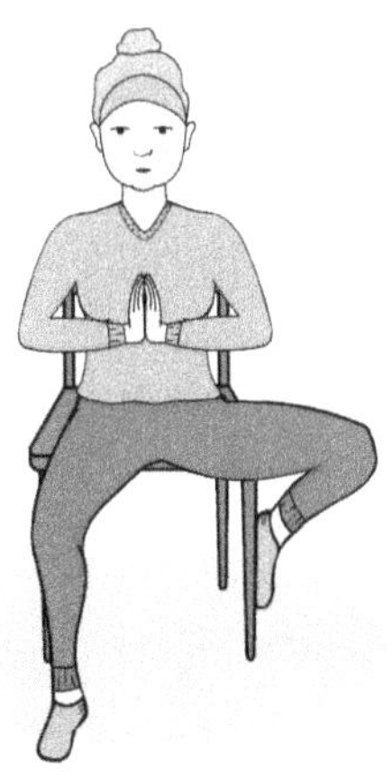

13

Chair Tree
Hold 3 breaths and switch sides.

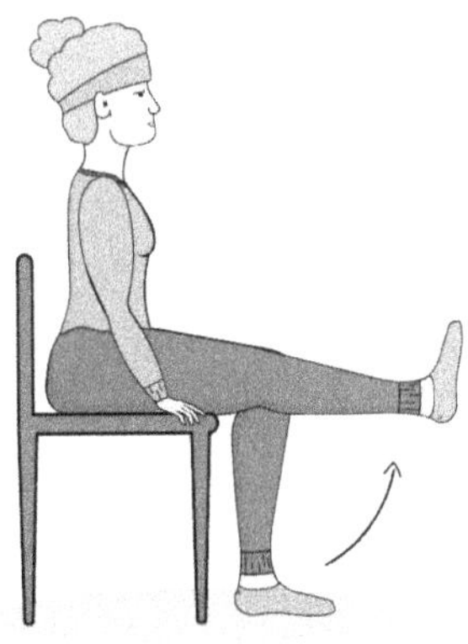

19

Seated Leg Extension
Hold 2 breaths and switch sides.
Repeat 4-times

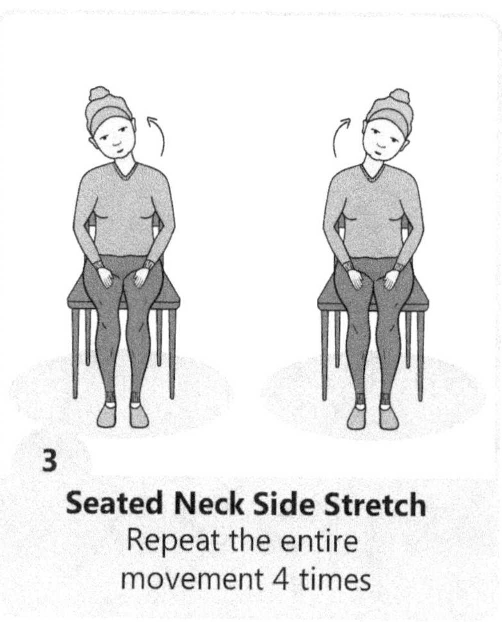

3

Seated Neck Side Stretch
Repeat the entire
movement 4 times

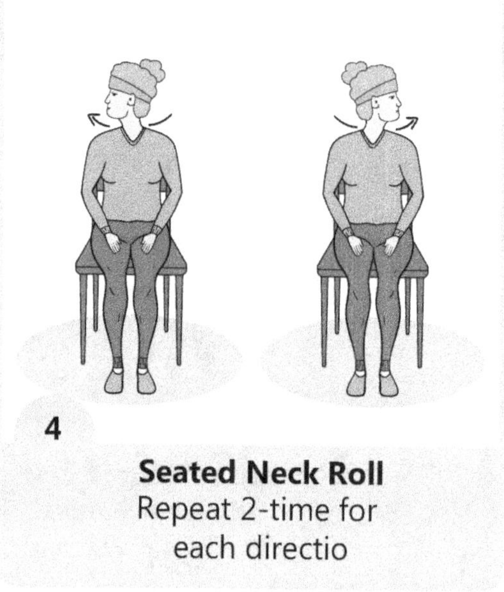

4

Seated Neck Roll
Repeat 2-time for
each directio

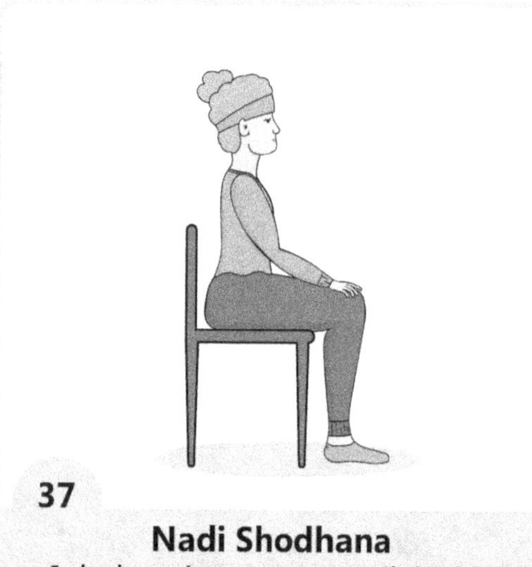

37

Nadi Shodhana
Inhale using one nostril, hold
and exhale using the other

Conclude your practice,
expressing gratitude aloud:

I am grateful for /to ...

Meditate (optional)

40

Savasana
Breathe, be grateful and
meditate.

CHAPTER 8: GENTLE ROUTINE FOR SENIORS WITH ACHY JOINTS AND MUSCLE STIFFNESS

This 10 to 15-minute gentle chair yoga routine is thoughtfully crafted to provide relief for seniors experiencing pain and discomfort, particularly those dealing with conditions like joint pain and muscle stiffness. The primary focus of this routine is to alleviate discomfort while promoting flexibility, strength, and relaxation. Key highlights of this routine include:

Joint Mobility: The routine aims to improve joint mobility, reducing stiffness and increasing overall comfort.

Muscle Flexibility: Gentle stretches help enhance muscle flexibility, further aiding in pain relief.

Strength Enhancement: While gentle, the routine includes exercises to maintain and strengthen muscle groups.

Holistic Well-Being: This routine promotes a holistic approach to well-being, addressing both physical and mental aspects of health.

It's always advisable to perform exercises that align with one's physical condition, and consulting a healthcare professional is recommended, especially for individuals with underlying health concerns.

Duration: 10 to 15 minutes

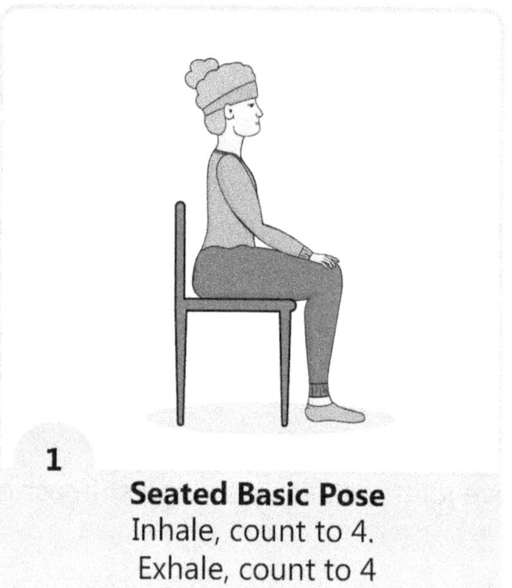

1

Seated Basic Pose
Inhale, count to 4.
Exhale, count to 4

Express your intention aloud starting with:

I intend to ...
I am ... (or)
I want to ...

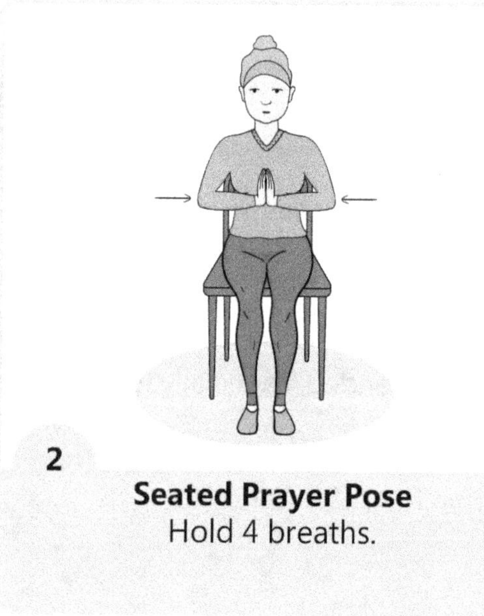

2

Seated Prayer Pose
Hold 4 breaths.

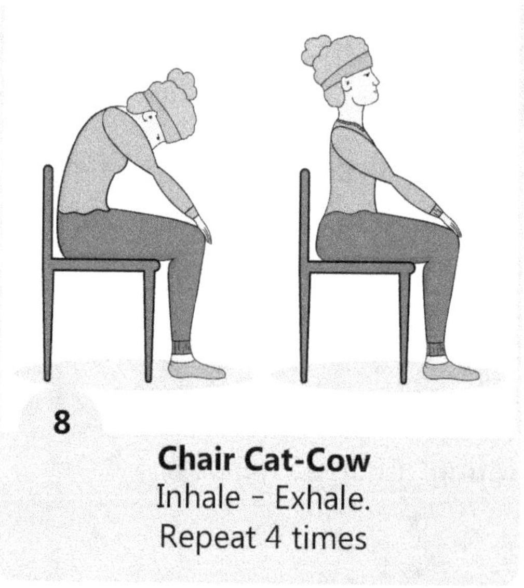

8

Chair Cat-Cow
Inhale – Exhale.
Repeat 4 times

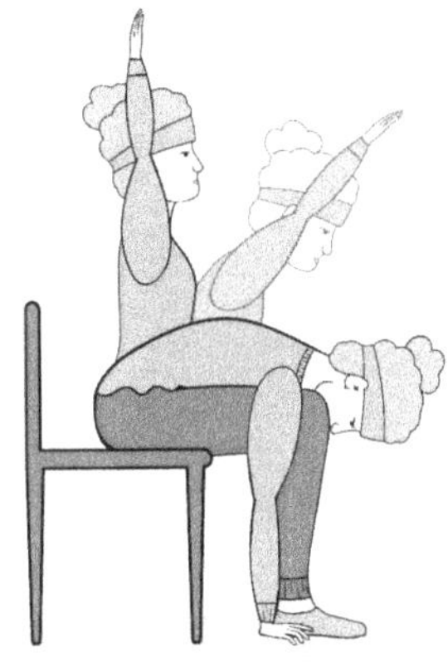

12

Seated Forward Fold

Hold 3 breaths and switch sides.
Repeat 4-times

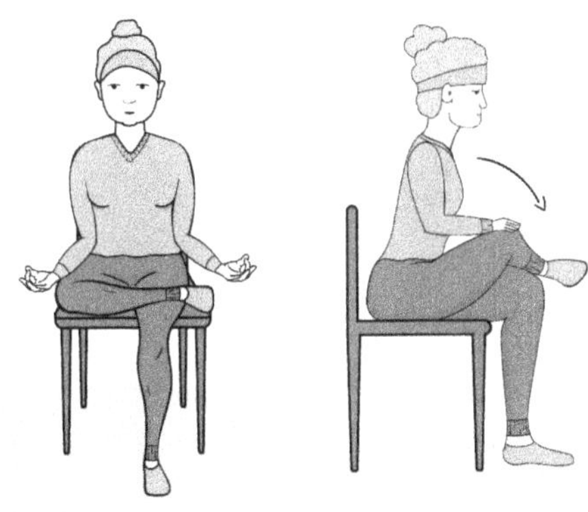

22

Chair Pigeon Pose

Hold 3 breaths and switch sides.

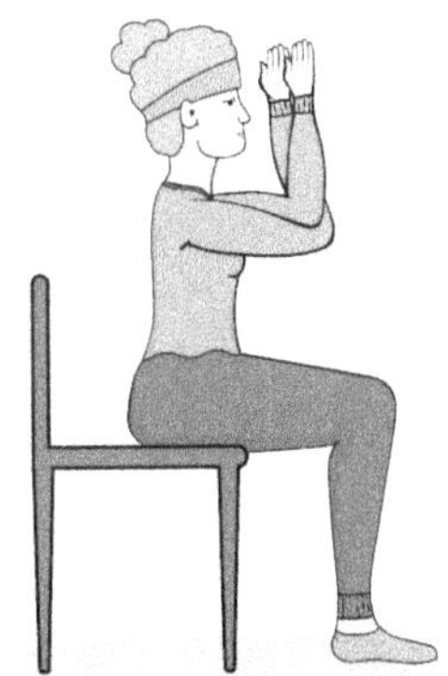

28

Seated Eagle Arms

Hold 4 breaths and switch sides.
Repeat 3 times.

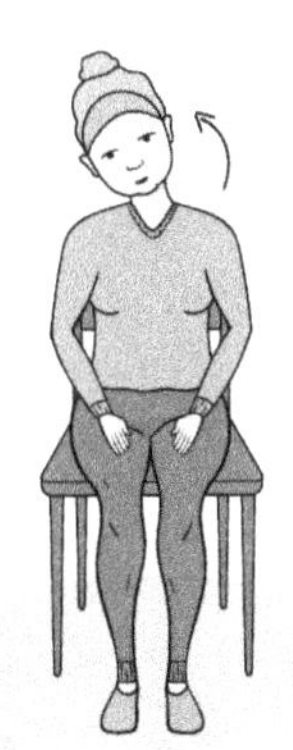

3

Seated Neck Side Stretch

Repeat the entire
movement 4 times

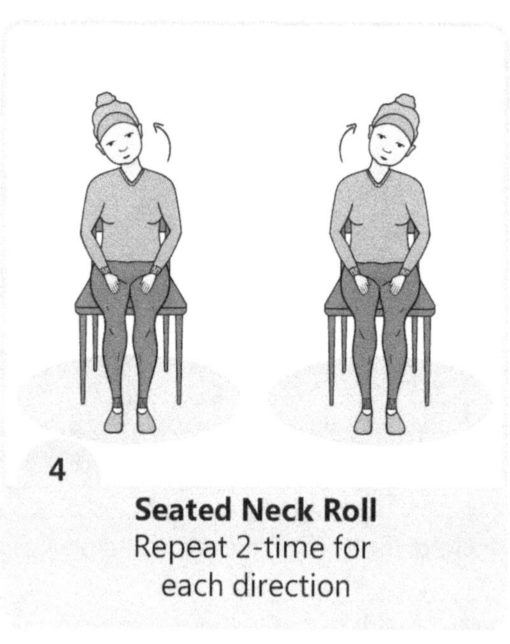

4

Seated Neck Roll
Repeat 2-time for
each direction

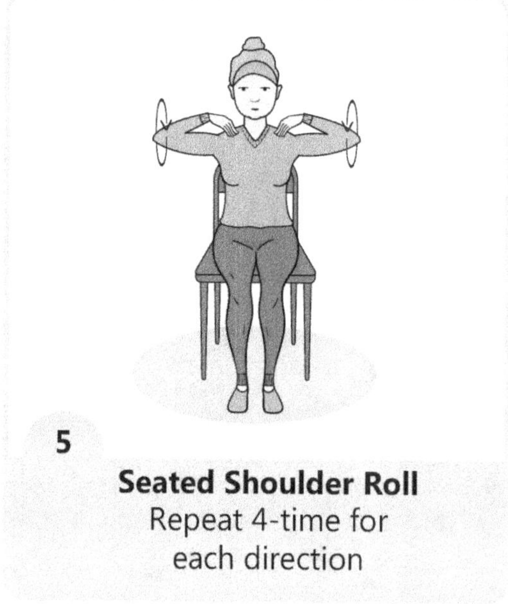

5

Seated Shoulder Roll
Repeat 4-time for
each direction

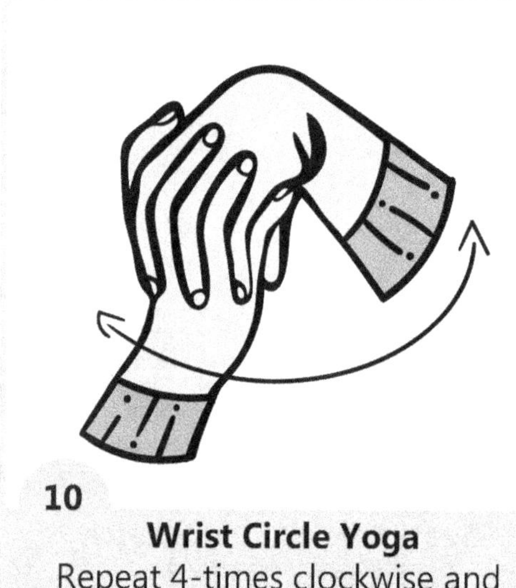

10

Wrist Circle Yoga
Repeat 4-times clockwise and
switch direction

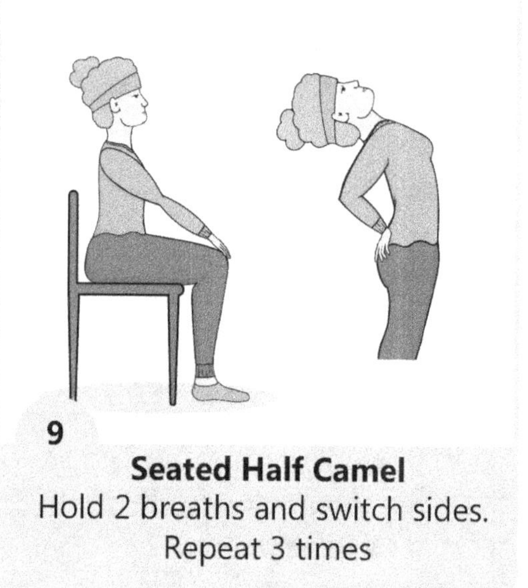

9

Seated Half Camel
Hold 2 breaths and switch sides.
Repeat 3 times

122

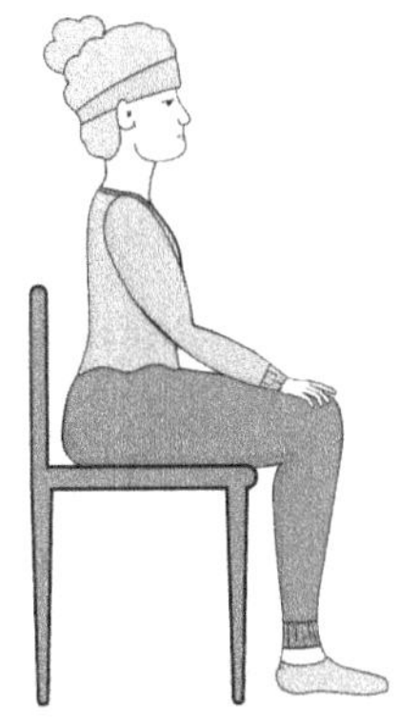

Conclude your practice,
expressing gratitude aloud:

I am grateful for /to ...

Meditate 5 minutes.

38

Samavriti Pranayama
Inhale -Hold – Exhale
Each step counting to 4. Repeat.

40

Savasana
Breathe, be grateful and
meditate.

CONCLUSION

Chair yoga is a safe and effective way for seniors to improve their overall health and well-being. Whether you want to lose weight, relieve pain, or gain mobility, these chair yoga routines provide step-by-step instructions and modifications for various abilities and conditions. By practicing regularly, you can enhance your physical and mental health, boost your confidence and independence, and reduce stress.

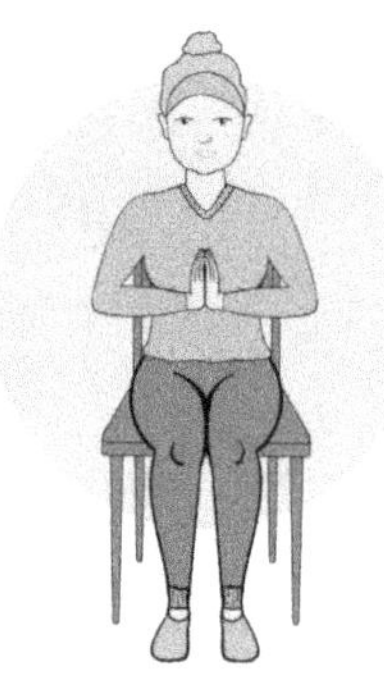

If you find this book helpful, consider leaving a review on Amazon. Your feedback helps us improve our products and services, inspires, and informs other seniors seeking to improve their health and quality of life through yoga.

Before you go, don't forget that by scanning the QR code below you will have instant access to 3 different eBooks.

1. 28-Day Chair Yoga Fitness Challenge
2. 15-Day Clean Eating Challenge
3. Audio Routines